CHRIS POWELL'S

CHOOSE MORE, LOSE MORE
FOR LIFE

ALSO BY CHRIS POWELL

Choose to Lose

CHRIS POWELL'S
CHOOSE MORE, LOSE MORE
FOR LIFE

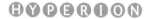

New York

Copyright © 2013 by Chris Powell

The credits on p. 289 constitute a continuation of this copyright page.

Library of Congress Cataloging-in-Publication Data has been applied for.

ISBN: 978-1-4013-2484-1

Book design by Chris Welch

FIRST EDITION

10 9 8 7 6 5 4 3 2 1

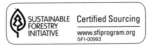

THIS LABEL APPLIES TO TEXT STOCK

We try to produce the most beautiful books possible, and we are also extremely concerned about the impact of our manufacturing process on the forests of the world and the environment as a whole. Accordingly, we've made sure that all of the paper we use has been certified as coming from forests that are managed, to ensure the protection of the people and wildlife dependent upon them.

To my amazing best friend, soul mate, coach, and wife, Heidi, who has been by my side from the beginning of this incredible journey. Everything within these pages we have learned, experienced, created, and completed, together. I insisted that the rest of this dedication be written by the both of us.

To our fathers, William Grant Powell and David Grant Lane: one still with us, and one smiling down from above.

You have both taught us some of the most valuable lessons in life. Thank you for teaching us that we are all human, and it's okay to struggle. You taught us that we are all perfectly imperfect, and that our challenges in life are blessings to make us stronger. Your examples of courage and vulnerability through your own trials continue to inspire us each and every day. You taught us that unconditional love is the most powerful thing in this world. Thank you for being our heroes.

Contents

Acknowledgments

This book, and the information, motivation, inspiration, and experience within it, could never have existed if it wasn't for the amazing team of people who have come together to make this all possible: Simon Green, Ryan Levine, Karl Austen, Constance Jones, Bonnie Schroader, Matt Inman, and the entire talented Hyperion team.

Thank you to my family, whose love and support over the years has carried me through my toughest times. I wouldn't be where I am without you.

Thank you to our transformation "Peeps." Without your courage to allow Heidi and me into your lives, to share openly and authentically, we could never have learned from one another. Our lives have forever been changed and enriched because of you, and for that we cannot begin to express enough our gratitude and appreciation.

Thank you to our team behind the camera: the production crew, trainers, coaches, therapists, counselors, and doctors who have come together to unconditionally support and brilliantly document our peeps' astonishing journey through a year of their transformation.

Thank you to our network, ABC, who has believed in our vision and given us a platform to share these inspiring stories of hope and change with the millions who desperately need them.

And thank YOU. Thank you for believing that change is possible. The power that we have within, to believe, is the rare human phenomenon that *we* believe in. That is what keeps us going. Belief is the magic that makes everything possible, and makes us all extraordinary.

CHRIS POWELL'S

CHOOSE MORE, LOSE MORE
FOR LIFE

SUCCESS STORY #1
OUR STORY

The story behind this book is the story of my life so far, which is truly a lesson in *choosing more*. But it's also the story of my life partnership with my wife and best friend, Heidi. As individuals and as a couple we choose to be on a continuous path toward positive transformation and growth, and through the trials and tribulations we guide each other as best we can. This makes my story *our* story, which is Success Story #1 in this book. I want to share it with you so you can see that you can experience the same success in your life that we've been so fortunate to have in ours. By *choosing* to transform yourself into the best possible you, you can write your own story of fulfillment. Your incredible voyage to transformation can begin right now; it starts with making a personal commitment to making your quality of life better by getting healthy and fit—and to dropping all those extra pounds (and the emotional weight) you're carrying around!

My story begins when I was fourteen, living with my family in Portland, Oregon. I was a frustrated athlete and a target for bullies because I'd always been the smallest kid in school. One day, my parents bought me a weight set, and I chose to transform my life. I built my muscles and became one of the strongest kids in my school, even though I was still the smallest.

Changing my body changed me—my whole identity—fundamentally. I became fascinated with fitness and the way it can transform not just your body but your life, so in college I chose to major in exercise science and learned all about how the human body works. When I graduated, I became a personal trainer and found my passion for helping other people lose weight and feel better about themselves. I started building a reputation as a fitness expert, making regular appearances on local TV in Phoenix, Arizona.

But by 2008 I'd gotten into business difficulties and lost almost everything I'd worked for. Things were so bad that I was living in my car. That's when my journey with my wife, Heidi, began. We first met on December 5, 2008, to be exact. Heidi was down on her luck, too: She'd gone through a divorce the year before and was fighting her own tough battles as a single mother raising two young kids. For both of us, life's slate had been wiped clean. We were ready for a major change.

I chose to try to figure out who I was, where I was headed, and why I had such a destructive past. I dove into self-help books and life-coaching seminars. During a lunch break of one of these seminars, I saw an absolutely beautiful woman. Boy, was she toned! I went up to her and told her that her arms looked amazing. I swear it wasn't a line (though at first she thought it was)—I really wanted to know how she was so fit. She'd been athletic all her life, had gotten certified as a personal trainer when she was nineteen, and had been weight training and playing sports for a long time. We obviously had a lot in common, and as two passionate trainers, conversation sparked up.

But we didn't flirt or try to impress each other—at that point in our lives, neither of us wanted the stress of a relationship. I was focused on figuring myself out, on sorting out why my life was where it was, on digging down to my foundation. Heidi was there for the same reason. When the seminar ended, we kept on talking for the rest of the evening. We were incredibly open, honest, and vulnerable with each other. What a cool way to start a friendship! Our connection was about . . . connecting—and about unconditional appreciation and acceptance of how perfectly imperfect we were.

In the months that followed, each of us had begun to regain our happiness in life, and we were enjoying our friendship so much. But we kept each other strictly in the "friend box." We e-mailed and texted and got together for lunch on a regular basis. I gave Heidi exercise and diet advice, and she gave me business and financial advice. As hard-core fitness buffs, we also grew closer as we worked out together. Our awesome friendship blossomed, and we helped each other put the pieces of our lives back together.

In the spring of 2009 I asked Heidi to come to work with me. She helped me out with my business and collaborated on developing the transformation paradigm. Together, we built a website, wrote magazine articles, and produced TV segments to bring the promise of transformation to a wide audience. We became true partners, equal contributors to the nutritional, training, and psychological underpinnings—the very definition—of life transformation. We were passionate about the work and driven to make a difference. It was exhilarating to work and dream together.

Great things started happening. I was back in my groove as a personal trainer and back on local TV. Then everything really took off. Back in 2003 I'd helped a client make an amazing transformation. A fantastic guy named David Smith had asked me to help him lose some weight—a lot of weight. When he came to me, he weighed more than 630 pounds. Twenty-two months later, he weighed 230 pounds. I had coached David to a 400-pound weight loss in two years!

Six years later, David's story had gone viral online, and the media had gotten wind of his astounding transformation. Some magazines in the UK picked it up, and then a British production company approached me about making a documentary. Before long, David and I appeared on *Oprah* and *20/20*. The *Today* show interviewed us. In July 2009, the TLC cable network aired *The 650-Pound Virgin*, a documentary about David's story.

Heidi was in my corner 100 percent, but there was still no romance. She had kids, which absolutely terrified me. She was afraid that I was a bachelor who would never understand the stresses and demands of parenting. I was wrapped up in my vision rather than in the hope of settling down. Then one day she brought her daughter, Marley, over to spend time with her while she worked in the office. Amidst the chaos of our crazy workday, I stepped back for the first time to watch her with her daughter. The moment I witnessed her relationship with her, how beautiful it was, it knocked me on my butt. This breathtaking woman had been right in front of me all along. It was the most powerful moment of clarity. I told Heidi I was head over heels, and it turned out she felt the same way! But it took a couple of months to convince her I was ready to take on parenthood! On June 30, 2010, we got married.

I became Dad to two great little kids, Matix and Marley, who showed me the ropes of being a parent. They've taken me to a whole new level of being and given me a huge appreciation for what parents do as they try to guide their kids in the right direction and help them lay a solid foundation for their lives. Heidi's guided my learning process and shown me how to create a culture of health and wellness in our family. And she's opened my eyes to how full and beautiful life can be with a family.

As our friendship and marriage have grown, Heidi and I have continued to *choose* personal transformation into the best "we" we can be (and we definitely have to work at it!). I wish I could say that only wonderful things have happened for us, but we've had our share of tough times. To

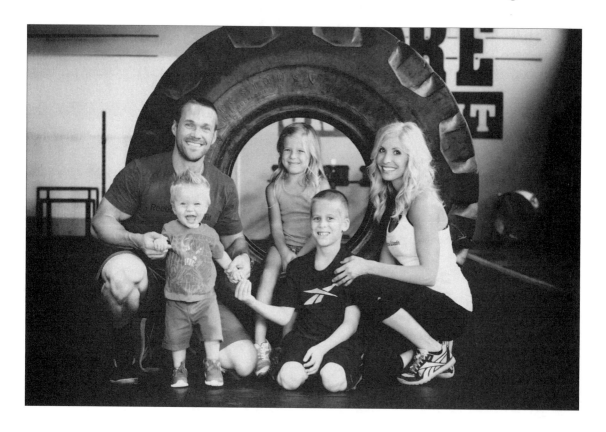

us, though, life's challenges—the bumps in the road—help us see the brilliance in what we do have, and they encourage us to grow as people. If life was all butterflies and roses, we wouldn't appreciate their beauty . . . and to be honest, it would be pretty darn boring!

But let's get back to the good stuff. On the phone one day, when I was catching up with a friend who works for a production company in Los Angeles, I mentioned that Heidi and I were bringing some clients to Arizona to coach them through weight-loss and life transformations. My friend told her boss about it, and twenty-four hours later she asked me to come to L.A. for a meeting.

In about a month with the creative folks in L.A., Heidi and I hammered out the concept for a television show for people to transform their lives by losing weight and embracing a healthy lifestyle. Then we went home, kept transforming clients, and continued building the business. We went on as usual. It all changed a couple of months later, when I got a phone call from the production company's CEO. ABC had picked up our show! In a matter of weeks I packed my bags and hit the road to make *Extreme Makeover: Weight Loss Edition*.

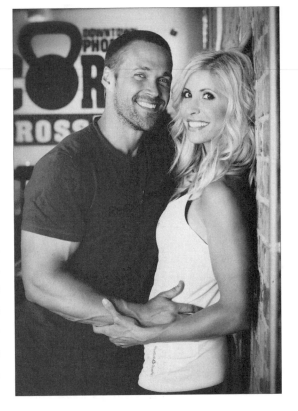

Season 1 premiered a month before our first wedding anniversary, and two weeks before our first child together, Cash, was born. Unbelievable, when only two and a half years ago both of us were at our all-time personal lows! The show was a mega-success, so ABC brought it back for Season 2 and then for Season 3. To support the show, Heidi and I created our Arizona Boot Camp, where participants who are struggling with their process can come for a week or two—or three, or more—to get Heidi's guidance through their transformation. So the transformations that you see on *Extreme Makeover* are truly a family affair: While I'm out on the road helping people on their home turf, Heidi's working with them in Arizona.

Doing the ABC show has been an awesome opportunity to work side by side with my best friend and wife. We bounce ideas off each other and come up with different tactics and approaches for helping each participant through his or her process. Early in 2012, Dr. Oz—the man behind *The Dr. Oz Show*—asked Heidi and me to be regular contributors on the show. More and more television and radio shows, websites, magazines, and newspapers have asked us to pass our insight along to their audiences.

It seems like a long, long time since that day in 2008 when Heidi and I were both so low and both searching for ourselves. Today, I know that even though we all *fall* sometimes, like I did before I met Heidi, it doesn't mean we *fail*. We *can* get up and keep going. I've learned not to listen when people tell me—or life tells me—no. I keep believing and keep going. It's part of my own ongoing transformation.

Our story is Success Story #1. I've been so fortunate to have Heidi as my true partner in the personal and professional learning experience that each day holds. Everything that happens in our lives presents an opportunity to discover wonderful new things about ourselves and about growing. *Our* philosophy of transformation—which goes way beyond weight loss and wellness—continues to evolve with every single person we coach.

As we learn and understand more and more about fitness and transformation, our goal is to give each new client a hand up not only to *lose* unwanted pounds, but to *choose* his or her own unique path to personal transformation. Now I'd like to empower you to choose to lose. I hope to be your partner in weight loss and life transformation: I'm so excited to share our philosophy with you and can't wait to help you write your own success story!

1

INTRODUCTION

There are thousands of diet and exercise programs around, and everyone's looking for "the right program for me." Somehow, only a few of us ever find it. Sure, plenty of diet plans melt the fat, but that's always going to happen when you take in fewer calories than you burn off. So everyone's convinced that this formula is all they need to know in order to get a permanently perfect body: diet + exercise = weight loss. Technically, that's correct. But the truth is that it's the magic inside you—what happens in your heart and mind—that makes weight loss happen! It's what turns weight loss into *life transformation*.

There are lots of ways to drop pounds and get in shape. But most of them take buckets of blood, sweat, and tears. No wonder we're always searching in the wrong place for a better weight-loss solution! I want to show you a different, easier, awesomely effective way to reach your weight and fitness goals, whatever they are. Whether you're going for a killer body or peak athletic performance or great overall health, this book will satisfy your needs. And I'm going to get you there in *the least amount of time, with the least amount of effort*.

Yawn. Every diet promises you'll get fantastic results with a minimum of work. Every diet guru says his or her scheme is different. How can I claim that my plan will do what all those others can't? To start with, I'm going to tell you to *stop thinking about food and stop thinking about exercise*—those are actually minor players in the weight-loss game!

In my eleven years as a personal trainer and fitness expert, I've learned something really big: *Dropping pounds and getting fit aren't really about diet and exercise.* I'm going to hand you the real keys to losing weight. When you read my clients' Success Stories and see the jaw-dropping transformations that they've achieved, you'll know my program works. And you'll wonder, "What do they know that I don't?"

The first and most important step is to *make a commitment to yourself* not just to lose weight but to change your life. On the day I start working with a client, we have a conversation that lays bare the truth behind the client's weight issues and reveals what the client really wants—and what the client actually can have. For most people I work with, this conversation is the turning point when they realize that transformation is a genuine possibility for them. That's why they go on to achieve such extraordinary results.

I can't say it enough: Reaching your weight and health goals, as well as staying healthy and gorgeous once you get there, is about transformation—remodeling your lifestyle, your life, and yourself! Yeah, trimming those excess inches can improve your life to some extent. But it really works the other way around: Transforming your life is *the key to getting lean* permanently and maintaining that fabulous body. What does transformation really mean, and how can you do it? Stick with me, and I'll show you.

Working with one amazing client after another, and working nonstop on myself to become the best me I can be, I've witnessed and experienced transformation. And I have uncovered the most crucial and powerful ingredients in transformation. They're just as important as—no, *more* important than—the physical techniques!

Here's the big news: Exploring your identity, *finding your authentic self,* and getting to know your emotional side—what makes you tick and what makes you stumble—are essential to transformation. So are believing that you can do it, keeping your promises to yourself, learning to bounce back from setbacks, and surrounding yourself with people who believe in you. I'd like to share all of this with you—that's why I wrote this book.

In my first book, *Choose to Lose: The 7-Day Carb Cycle Solution,* I laid out a terrific diet system called *carb cycling,* and I introduced a super-easy workout method that amplifies carb cycling's weight-loss impact and accelerates the get-fit process. I taught people how to integrate basic carb cycling and simple ten-minute exercise routines into their lives so they could put the 7-Day Carb Cycle Solution to work—for real. But I recognize that no exercise program is one-size-fits-all. Now I want to show you how to work the program in the way that's best for *you*!

You'll find indispensable basics and a solid foundation for carb cycling in *Choose to Lose*, but even if you didn't read my first book, this one will rock your world! See, this book gives you the advanced version of the info in the first one, and *turbocharges* it. I've taken what I've learned about carb cycling, exercise, and transformation in the past couple years and added it to the mix. That's loads of learning, because the people who used my first book had incredible success slimming down and improving their lives.

After reading *Choose to Lose,* thousands of people embraced the carb-cycle lifestyle, and the results speak for themselves. I've been overwhelmed by the crowds of people who've told me that they can't believe how miraculously carb cycling helped them finally lose ten, fifty, even two hundred pounds. Many of them were finally able to break through weight plateaus they had always struggled with! Their stories of transformation have opened my eyes again and again.

I've peppered this book with wonderful testimonials from people who have *changed their lives* through our methods of transformation and carb cycling. I know you'll be blown away by these stories—not only by the incredible weight-loss and fitness achievements, but by the life transformations these people have made from unhappiness, frustration, and loneliness to self-fulfillment, joy, and success.

Seeing the benefits that so many people have gotten from carb cycling, it's my responsibility to reach out to more folks with my upgraded system—and to help those who've already started stay on their paths to lifelong fitness. In this book you'll find *even more* inspiration and guidance, more personal inventories and logs, new nutritional and workout options, and a whole new slew of easy, delicious recipes. There's even a quiz to help you pick the best plan for you. If you're a newbie, you'll be able to hit the ground running not only with the short version of the basics but with the advantage of the enhancements I've made! You'll thank thousands of confirmed carb cyclers for sharing their experiences as you choose more and lose more for life!

One thing I learned from the e-mails and letters I've received is that some people find the principles of carb cycling and general nutrition kind of complex at first, and that it takes some time for some of them to figure out how to turn the facts into action. So this book is a lot more interactive and better at helping you to bridge the gap between its pages and your actual life. It's packed with step-by-step advice and all kinds of tools that make carb cycling real, hands-on, and practical. I'm going to introduce you to *a truly doable, livable, and sustainable weight-loss and weight-maintenance program*. You're going to love my fast, easy, and convenient techniques!

Whatever your specific situation, the foundation of the nutrition section of this book is: *There's a carb cycle for that*. You can adjust the carb-cycle plans, workouts, and recipes according to your needs and to the demands of your life. *Customization* puts you in control, because all of the techniques can work for you no matter where you are in your life and in your transformation process! You'll have the flexibility you want.

I introduced my *Classic Cycle* in my first book. It's the simplest of the four carb cycles laid out in this book, although it's not the easiest. All those carb cyclers who read *Choose to Lose* started their weight-loss journey with the Classic Cycle, and the ones who've stuck with it have lost weight quickly and steadily. If you're ready to take on a moderate challenge but like your path straight and smooth, my good old Classic Cycle will reward you with fast weight loss.

The *Easy Cycle* is a laid-back version of the Classic Cycle. I've designed it for people who are just starting their journey and who feel like they might lack the willpower to stick with carb cycling. It's especially for you if you need to reward yourself regularly with your favorite foods. It's for you if you're terrified to take the first steps toward transformation because you don't want to feel deprived and restricted. If you do the Easy Cycle with no deviations, you will succeed, because it's built around idea that *if you can't have it today, you can have it tomorrow*. You're allowed to cheat every other day, but you'll still cut your calories in half! Of course, you won't lose pounds as fast as on the other two plans in the book, but you *will* get instant gratification from instant results. You'll find that the Easy Cycle is a truly sustainable lifestyle program that just about anyone can do. It is the easiest way to start your transformation journey.

Then there's the *Turbo Cycle*, which accelerates and intensifies your carb-cycling results so you can reach your weight-loss goals as quickly as possible. If you're really antsy to get there and you're ready to take on a big commitment, this is the cycle for you. It's carb cycling, turbocharged. The Turbo Cycle revs up your carb cycle so *you get results faster* than with the Classic Cycle or the Easy Cycle. It maximizes weight loss by including more fat-burning days than the other plans do. And I've scheduled metabolism-boosting days strategically, to prime your body to burn more effectively on your fat-burning days. How cool is that?

The *Fit Cycle* is for you if you're already super-active but you want to drop some weight. Even though you burn a lot of calories and need a lot of carbs, you can still carb cycle to lose weight and avoid gaining new fat. The Fit Cycle allows you to lose a lot of weight while keeping your carb intake high to fuel your performance, even if you work out or compete five or six days a week. With the Fit Cycle, you can actually *increase your performance* while maximizing the weight-loss benefits of carb cycling. This plan is so fantastic that I continue to use it. I'm carb cycling for life!

So whoever you are, whatever your strengths and weaknesses, wherever you're headed, *there's a carb cycle for that*. But I know you want it to be as easy and convenient as possible, to fit into your hectic life. How can I make the program work for you as you face everyday reality? You're busy, you've got a crazy schedule, you spend a lot of your time out of the house, you have only so much time to focus on the carb-cycling nutrition plan. So you've got challenges. How can you pull it off?

I'm going to give you recipes, meal plans, and eating tips that make the carb-cycle diet superconvenient. I'll lay out more than *thirty* delicious recipes that you can make in less than five minutes. I'll also give you high- and low-carb variations on these recipes so that you have more than sixty delicious meals to choose from! *Preparing your food will be quick and easy, and your meals will be cheap.* Throw "I can't afford to eat healthy" out the window. In fact, you can't afford *not* to eat healthy! And you *can* eat healthy on the carb-cycle program, because you can *customize* it to your needs. It will be easier than ever to eat right—which means you'll succeed in your weight-loss goals.

"Okay," you say, "I kinda get it. But didn't you say something about exercise, too?" Yes, to really maximize what carb cycling can do for you, you'll need to *get your body moving*. You'll need to burn the carbs that are stored in your muscles and jack your metabolism to the roof by developing and moving those muscles. Sounds intense, right? And time-consuming. Well, actually, not so much.

I've designed simple *muscle-developing* workouts that I call *Shapers* because they sculpt your body. In this book I've included twenty brand-new ones I call "9-Minute Missions" because you can complete them in just nine minutes. You'll begin every weekday by completing a 9-Minute Mission—the ultimate way to start your day! For cardio fitness, I've designed *muscle-moving* workouts that I call *Shredders* because they burn fat like crazy. Shredders are less intense than Shapers and take a little bit longer to do—anywhere from ten to sixty minutes, according to your fitness level. (If you're super-fit and want to get fitter, you can make your Shredder workouts even longer.) I ask you to do Shredders five days a week. You can take both the Shapers and Shredders laid-back and easy or rigorous and demanding, depending on whether you're just starting out, a weekend golfer, or a marathon runner. To help you fit the workouts into your day, and to help you stick with them, *I've made the exercises easy, effective, and fun*. Really—it's true!

The Shapers and Shredders are easy because they're based on the types of movement that your body does naturally. Every day you push (closing your car door), pull (opening your dishwasher), crunch (sitting up in bed), and squat (sitting down at your desk). I'm not asking you to do anything that you don't already do! This is part of what makes the workouts so effective—this, and because you'll be doing *lots of different exercises*, not the same thing over and over from day to day.

I'll teach you many variations on the Shapers and Shredders, and I've created a whole month of different workouts for you. Changing it up like this makes the workouts fun because you don't get bored. And the most fun is that *the Shapers and Shredders get results*. When you repeat your

9-Minute Missions the following month, you'll experience a significant and noticeable increase in your fitness. It's awesome!

But back to the basics: Weight loss isn't just about diet and exercise—it's about transformation! In the chapters that follow you'll get to know yourself and your goals, and find out what it means to transform your life. I'll let you in on *the secrets to transforming* and on the importance of personal integrity and keeping your promises to yourself.

You'll find inspiration and validation in the stories of other carb cyclers who have reached their goals or who are still struggling to get there. Fellow carb cyclers will show you what to expect on the journey to transformation, and will reassure you that, even if you stumble along the way, *you can fall without failing* on your path to a great physique and a great life!

You don't have to understand all this transformation stuff before you start carb cycling; I guarantee you'll come to understand it along the way. Bottom line, this book is *a call to action*. If you want results—if you want to lose that weight and transform your life—you need to stop thinking about it and get going! You hold in your hand the map to an incredible path to success, and *I'll be right beside you 100 percent*, cheering you all the way to your finish line. You're choosing to make a healthy change, and *I'm choosing you*. It's going to be a wonderful journey for both of us!

Like it says on the cover, we're doing this *for life*!

2

THE TRUE SECRET OF
TRANSFORMATION

Tony was always overweight, even as a kid. No wonder: All his life he used food as a replacement for the love and joy he never had.

When he was four years old, Tony's alcoholic parents abandoned him, handing him off to relatives. His mother showed up sometimes and dragged him into her life of bar-hopping and one-night stands. Soon she tossed Tony back to his relatives for good, and they passed him around, arguing over who would "get" him—and his welfare checks—next.

Tony turned to food for relief and comfort. He didn't get to eat very often, so whenever he had the chance he ate as much as he could. Finally, when he was fourteen, Tony ran away, stuffing his possessions into a garbage bag and finding a room for $50 a month. Following his stomach, he got a job at a fast-food restaurant, where he wolfed down the free burgers and fries. If he wasn't at work, he didn't eat—and he only felt safe when his belly was full.

Things started looking better when he got married, but then his son was born severely handicapped. Tony walled out the emotional stress with food. He started yo-yo dieting, losing ten pounds, gaining fifteen back, dropping fifteen then gaining thirty, and so on, eventually eating himself all the way to 438 pounds. His bulk earned him the nickname "Big Guy."

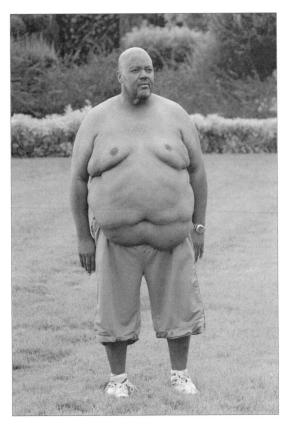

Tony before

As Tony's weight went up, his quality of life went downhill. He couldn't function normally, and he was sick, tired, depressed, and embarrassed about his appearance. Then he went for a physical and the doctor told him that he was not just overweight: He was morbidly obese. In the process of killing his pain with food, Tony was killing himself.

At the age of forty-nine, Tony realized that something had to give, and he didn't want it to be his heart. He tried exercising, but he was never able to stick with it. He knew he needed help if he was ever going to get fit. That's when my producers at *Extreme Makeover: Weight Loss Edition* heard about him and invited him onto the show.

Tony's goal was to lose at least two hundred pounds. What he didn't realize at first was that it would take a lot more than exercising and eating right to do it. But then Heidi and I introduced him to the power of transformation. I spoke with Tony about my own experiences with homelessness and despair. I told him I was proud of him for taking on the biggest challenge of his life. He began to understand that I believed in him.

When he felt how deeply I believed in him, Tony started to believe in himself for the first time in his life. He began by believing he could drop the weight. And he did: By his six-month weigh-in on the show, he had lost 156 pounds. Then, seven months into his weight-loss journey, he experienced *the moment of clarity* that's essential to successful transformation. It's the moment when he understood down to his core why he'd been driven to gain weight, and what being overweight meant for him; when he truly accepted that he *wanted* to change and that change was in his total control.

As his fat melted away, he couldn't hide behind his weight anymore. He decided it was time to deal with his past, once and for all. He realized that he wasn't just a Big Guy: He was a person named Tony, and he wanted to be proud of himself. He believed that he could love himself.

Not only was Tony incredibly motivated to lose his excess pounds, he was determined to lose all the other heavy baggage he'd been lugging around all his life. He began to understand that he'd spent his whole life eating his emotions and fears, and his anger at his parents. Bottling up his feelings had always brought him down—and made him eat. When he realized this about his past and himself, Tony knew he had to become completely honest with himself and others.

Once he opened up to the people who supported him, Tony had even more faith in himself. He came to believe that he deserved to be happy and loved. Powered by his self-confidence, he kept losing weight and healing emotionally—and learning who he really was. Now Tony knows that he's not defined by the times in life that he falls, but by the times when he gets back up.

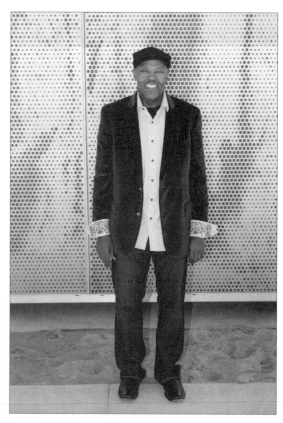

Tony after

Heidi and I are still inspired by Tony's unshakable belief in himself, which launched him into one of the most awesome transformations we've ever witnessed. Like Tony, you can radically transform your life if you believe in yourself. That's what will empower you to lose that weight and become the person you dream of being. Once you believe, you have taken the first step on your transformation journey.

One of our all-time favorite sayings goes something like this: "Dare to dream. For your dreams become words, your words become actions, your actions become habits, your habits become character, and your character becomes your destiny." That's the truth we see in Tony's story, and that's the truth that will make you a fantastic success!

The Meaning of Transformation

The real key to fulfilling your weight-loss dreams isn't diet or exercise: It's *life transformation*. Sure, you'll need to eat right and burn more calories to get the body you want, but that's secondary.

So what is transformation? It's not something you can measure, like the pounds on your scale or the inches around your waist. It's something you feel. When Heidi and I first meet our clients, we ask, "How do you feel about yourself?" Almost every one of them answers, "I hate myself. Look how I've allowed myself to get to three hundred, four hundred, five hundred, six hundred pounds! Why wouldn't I hate myself?" Then we ask them, "But why do you *really* hate yourself?" Most of them say something like "I'm a compulsive overeater. I don't have the willpower to exercise. I'm pathetic!" They don't see what's really going on, and they don't understand how it happened.

You don't have to be obese to feel this way. You might be struggling to lose fifteen or thirty pounds, or even just those last five pounds, and you're not getting anywhere. You think you're a failure. "I'm weak and worthless," you say. "Just look at me—I'm fat. I'm just an out-of-shape disappointment."

Like my obese clients, you're certain that you hate yourself because you're overweight, and you're certain that you're overweight because you eat too much. But in fact, you've got it backward. You eat too much and you're overweight *because you hate yourself.* You don't believe in yourself and you don't know how to love yourself. If you want to get the body you dream of, this needs to change. You need to transform from the inside out.

Transformation isn't weight loss: *It's your journey toward loving yourself.* It's about growing your self-esteem, accessing your inner power, and building your sense of self-worth. That's the magic that can energize ordinary people—including you—to do extraordinary things. And one of those things is to finally, permanently drop those pounds.

After our clients reach their goal weight, and even while they're still working at it, they realize that their journey *isn't about that number on the scale*. When they've tapped into their extraordinary potential and made themselves their first priority, they hold their chins high, square their shoulders, and puff their chests out, because they love themselves! They're proud of their beautiful new bodies, but they're even more thrilled that they've dug themselves out of their emotional hole and transformed their lives.

Their self-hatred is gone and their self-esteem has shot up to stratospheric heights. It blows us away every single time we see our clients leave behind defeat and hopelessness to reach victory and self-love. I know that *you can make that transformation, too!*

Secrets of Transformation

I'm going to let you in on a few fundamental secrets that make lifelong transformation possible. Thanks to real-life experience with our awesome clients and trial and error in our own lives, Heidi and I have been fortunate to gain so much insight into how transformation happens. In this book I want to share four phenomenal and powerful things that we have discovered are *absolutely essential to every single transformation.*

Deep inside, you already know these four secrets—in fact, you're driven by them. You just haven't deciphered the code . . . yet. Once you truly absorb these secrets and put them into action, the physical nuts and bolts of carb cycling will fall into place. You will, for the first time in your life, completely understand what went wrong with every single diet you've tried. These secrets put lifelong transformation and carb-cycling success within your reach. Use them, and I *know* you'll make it.

The First Secret: Believe

I've always said that belief is the magic ingredient: When we *believe we can*, we tap into our extraordinary human ability to persevere, and we put forth the effort required to get us to our destination. This secret might sound so simple (because it is): *Believe in yourself,* believe in this process, and believe that your transformation is possible. Not just transformation of your body, but lifelong transformation of yourself. If you don't at least believe "maybe I can," then transformation isn't going to happen for you. But when you believe transformation is possible, it is.

With belief, you're capable of accomplishing things you never before thought you could do. You tap into extraordinary inner power that gives you the drive and perseverance you need to get going and keep going, day in and day out, to lose that weight and to change your life. *Belief gives you the power to achieve the extraordinary!*

But believing in yourself can also be complicated. As Henry Ford once stated, "Whether you think you can or you can't, you're right." Millions upon millions of people have attempted and failed and attempted and failed to slim down, and they don't believe in themselves anymore. What if you're in such a dark place of self-hatred that you don't see how you could ever believe in yourself? Is your situation hopeless? No, it really isn't. *It's okay if you don't believe in yourself yet.* Don't worry: I'll show you the way. I'll teach you what Heidi and I have learned about growing your belief in yourself—the steps are very simple. No matter how discouraged and desperate you are, you can learn the steps. When you do, nothing will be able to stop you!

WHY WE WORK WITH SUPER-OBESE CLIENTS

We know something you don't know: *We know what you're capable of*—because we've seen what truly challenged people are capable of. It's something we've learned by working with extremely obese people who are so discouraged, so low in life that they've lost hope. They come from a place of such despair and darkness that a life of health and happiness seems like an untouchable dream. They don't believe in themselves, but right when we start working with them Heidi and I let them know that *we believe in them*. We show them the secrets to growing their self-belief.

One reason we choose to work with people who face the longest transformation journeys is to prove over and over again that transformation is possible. If they can do it, so can you! I've filled this book with the amazing stories of some of our obese clients so you can witness the power of believing. I hope that when you read these you'll experience a moment of clarity and say to yourself, "Oh my gosh! That's me! I get it now. If they can lose all that weight, I can, too. *I believe that I can!*" It's fantastic when that little light goes on in your head. Read on, and believe me, it will.

For starters, take a few minutes to reflect on and write down some of your past successes and accomplishments.

Seven great things that happened to me in the past year:
1.
2.
3.
4.
5.
6.
7.

Three people whose lives I've made significantly better (in any year):
1.
2.
3.

Three people who have made *my* life significantly better (in any year):
1.
2.
3.

What was my best day ever? Why was it so great?
....
....

What was the best-ever day of my career? Why was it so great?
....
....

What am I most happy about achieving in the past year? In my life?

....

....

What was the smartest decision I made in the past twenty-four months?

....

....

Who is my best friend? What makes our relationship so special?

....

....

Who's my biggest cheerleader when I set a goal?

....

....

What's the best compliment I ever received?

....

....

What's the most daring thing I've ever done?

....

....

What are my passions?

....

....

What are my skills and talents?

....

....

What do I love about my life right now? (List everything!)

....

....

What am I most grateful for?

....

....

Think about it: You've got a lot going for you!

The Second Secret: Keep Your Promises

You might think our obese clients reach their weight-loss goals one meal or one mile or one pound at a time. But in fact, they get there *one promise at a time*. Sure, eating right and working out are the physical reasons that they lose 250 pounds, drop 20 sizes, and shed 100 inches off their measurements. Good habits are what take down their cholesterol levels and make them healthy from the inside out. But each of these habits started as a commitment to making a small change in their daily routine. The real reason our clients make these incredible achievements is that *when they make a promise to themselves, they keep it.*

How do they do it? Our clients' promises have something in common: They become so strong that they're *virtually unbreakable*. When they stand tall at the end of their year-long journey, chest out and chin high, our clients celebrate the self-love that they've discovered and nurtured month after month. They couldn't care less about the fat-loss benefits of thirty minutes on the treadmill.

What they *do* care about is that they *promised* themselves thirty minutes, and completed the full thirty . . . maybe even an extra minute or two! They *never* stop at twenty-nine minutes. I repeat, NEVER. If they did, their self-esteem and self-belief would take huge body blows that could be devastating—and even spin them into a downward spiral.

But these fierce guys and gals weren't always so tough. Like you, they had to start somewhere. . . . That somewhere was *integrity*. Integrity—honoring your word—is an ideal in every society. Throughout history "a man of his word" has earned respect and admiration. Because of this, most of us are terrific at keeping promises to others. If we give someone our word, gosh darn it, we're going to keep our promise! But what about keeping your promises to the most valuable and important person in the world? What about *keeping your promises to you*?!

Listen up, because THIS IS THE KEY to transformation: *The more you honor your integrity, the more dignity you have.* Your promises to yourself must be so important and easily kept that you'll reach out and grab them every single day—because *you* want what you've promised yourself!

Keeping each promise to yourself has to be your focus, because it shows you that you are *your own top priority*. Each promise made is another step toward valuing and loving yourself, and a brick in the foundation of your transformation. Each promise kept—your integrity—is the mortar that holds the bricks together, and the more promises you honor, the stronger the foundation gets.

Every time you make a promise to yourself, your self-esteem is on the line, so make only first-class promises you know you can keep. Give yourself the respect you deserve by making honest and authentic ones. How many times have you made wishy-washy, halfhearted promises like "The diet starts Monday," or "I'll work out when I have the time"? And how many times have you shelved these pledges? Yeah, over and over and over again. You've got to get serious about your integrity. Transformation happens when you honor your promises over your reasons. So look yourself in the mirror; make a solid, real promise; and then fulfill that promise. The outcome will be powerful beyond measure.

THE PAIN OF BROKEN PROMISES

But the outcome of breaking a promise to yourself is devastating. When you promise yourself that you'll lose weight, and then break that promise, you might think at first, "Oh, well, no harm done—I'll try again." Well, guess what? *A lot* of harm was done!

Your diet's out the window. Another chance at transformation evaporates. But that's not the crux of the issue. If you break a promise—any promise—to yourself, you're *worse off* than if you'd never made that promise in the first place. When the day is over, the lights go out, and you're all alone, you're left with the shame of another failure. Either the negative self-talk begins or your bruised ego comes up with a million and one reasons why the diet didn't work this time: "I don't have time for breakfast!" "I broke a nail chopping vegetables!"

But the fact of the matter is that you broke a promise. It hurts, doesn't it? It undermines your self-esteem, your self-love, and your self-will. You nosedive right back to where you started, except this time you crash a little bit farther from your goals! Once again you think, "I knew I couldn't stick with it. I don't have what it takes." So guess what happens to that first trans-formation secret—*believing in yourself*? Any glimmer of belief you had fades to black, and your possibility for transformation crumbles.

WHY DO WE BREAK OUR PROMISES TO OURSELVES?

Right about now you're probably wondering, "How can I possibly keep my promises to myself all the time?" Yeah, life is busy. Life happens. And life isn't fair. You have to run the errands and pick the kids up from three different schools. Your spouse has to work late, so you've got to make sure the kids do their homework and their chores, and you've got your own chores to do. Before you know it, you're exhausted and you're ordering a pizza instead of prepping and steaming that batch of veggies. Oh yeah, and the thirty minutes of cardio you were going to do? Not going to hap-pen today. Your promises to yourself have flown out the window.

Let me tell you: There are promises, and then there are *promises*. There are promises that can be kept, and ones that can't. And it's not be-cause you're lazy or weak or insincere. Heidi and I have seen our clients break thousands of promises to themselves, and it's always painful, but we've discovered that most of those broken promises *were just out of whack*!

Some of the most out-of-whack promises our clients make are *inflated promises*. They make themselves a whole bunch of promises at once, or just one unnecessarily huge one. I can't tell you how many times we've heard people promise to do thirty minutes of cardio every morning, or to eat five smaller meals every day, or to never eat pizza again. No way! A few of them might succeed, but the majority are destined to fail. These promises are way too big!

Come to think of it, nearly every diet book and weight-loss program—including this one!—is a compilation of potentially inflated promises. At some point, you've probably made the mistake of jumping into a new diet and exercise plan full-bore, trying to make radical changes in your lifestyle right away. It almost *guarantees* you'll give up! Moving too fast and expect-ing too much of yourself, you end up breaking your promises to yourself. You might try to make yourself feel better by saying, "That diet's no good."

Maybe, maybe not. But that's not why your promises broke: They popped because they were inflated!

Do yourself—and your self-esteem, and your transformation—a huge favor and take it easy! Within these pages I offer a whole series of promises in the form of nutrition guidelines and exercise schedules that will *absolutely* give you the body you want. Each one is sound and levelheaded, but if you roll them all up into one giant promise, you've got quite a load to carry—and you're bound to drop it.

Don't get me wrong, I appreciate your enthusiasm, vigor, and desire to take it all on! But making too many promises at once just doesn't work. Believe me, you'll reach your goals—if you keep your feet on the ground. Believe in yourself by making promises you can keep!

Why do *you* break your promises to yourself? Do you sabotage yourself by making inflated promises? Think about it and write down the answers to these questions.

What were my New Year's resolutions last year? What other promises have I recently made to myself?

....

....

Did I keep any of them? Why or why not?

....

....

Did I make any progress on them? Why or why not?

....

....

Did I abandon them? Why or why not?

....

....

When I make a promise to myself, do I keep it? Why or why not?

....

....

When I make a promise, do I write it down? Post reminders everywhere?

....

....

Do I share my promises with anyone else? When I do, are they support-ive, or do they doubt I'll be able to keep them?

....

....

What's the biggest obstacle to keeping my promises to myself? Time? Money? Friends? Family? Anything else?

....

....

How can I plan ahead and work around these obstacles?

....

....

What will it take to make my promises to myself the number one pri-ority in my life?

....

....

THE POWER OF KEEPING YOUR PROMISES

As the old Chinese proverb goes, "Every journey begins with a single step." The way we see it, every transformation begins with a single prom-ise. That's why the very first transformation promise you make to your-self must be so small that it's actually attainable, even when life gets in the way. It has to be so doable that you know you can *fulfill it*. Then you can add another little promise and master that one. Each tiny promise is a step on your journey of transformation.

Here's an example: When people ask us how much cardio they should do to burn fat, our answer is "Gimme five minutes." Doesn't matter what it is—a jog around the block, walking in place while watching TV—just do it for five minutes. It's a five-minute promise that you can fulfill every day. If five minutes make you feel so good you want to do five more, that's great: You'll just reach your goal faster. But the promise is for only five minutes of cardio. Hit those five and you win. Period. Do four minutes and fifty-nine seconds and you lose. It's not about the cardio—it's about *you* and the *promise* you made! Get it yet?

Because it's so important to keep the promises you make to yourself, don't go overboard. Start slowly, by making *just one small promise*—"I will eat one serving of vegetables today," "I will take the stairs today." Every single promise puts your self-love on the line, so only make promises that you can keep—and keep them! I see the payoff for our clients: When they keep their promises, they learn how to love themselves, and they can do almost anything. Loving yourself is the *most valuable gift* you can give yourself. When you love yourself, you can realize your dreams.

THE POWER PROMISE

I want to give you every possible advantage in making your physical and emotional transformation, so I've written 101 basic, realistic promises that you can use (one at a time!) along the way. I call these the *Power Promises.* Each of these is a great place to start your transformation.

Take a look through the Power Promises. See how easy they are? If you make just one Power Promise to yourself, your chances of keeping it are incredibly good. So pick a promise and focus on keeping it. When you master it, add a second promise, make it happen, then a third . . . and so on. Give yourself as long as you need to fulfill each promise to yourself. By succeeding, you'll come to *believe* that you can transform your body and your life. Keeping your first promises to yourself will psych you up to *do this*!

The Power Promises fall into three categories that are central to transformation.

Food Promises—I Will:
1. Choose skim milk over whole milk.
2. Eat at least one serving of veggies every day.
3. Avoid drinks with refined sugar.
4. Cut out the beer and alcohol.
5. Drink half as many ounces of water daily as I weigh in pounds.
6. Drink water before each meal.
7. Use a smaller coffee cup.
8. Leave cream and sugar out of my coffee.

9. Eat breakfast every morning.
10. Eat low-sugar, high-fiber breakfast cereal.
11. Eat three meals and two snacks a day.
12. Set an alarm so I remember to eat every three hours.
13. Eat protein at every meal.
14. Quit grazing on junk food in the afternoon.
15. Keep healthy snacks on hand at home, work, and anywhere else I eat.
16. Stop eating my kids' food.
17. Brush my teeth after dinner so I don't eat later.
18. Stop eating after my fifth meal.
19. Pack each day's snacks and lunch in the morning, when I'm fresh and motivated.
20. Stop eating in the car.
21. Say no to fast food.
22. Put half of every restaurant meal in a take-out container before I start eating.
23. Eat from a salad plate instead of a dinner plate.
24. Eat slowly.
25. Occasionally enjoy my favorite foods in moderation so I don't feel deprived.
26. Stop eating off my friends' or spouse's plates.
27. Skip seconds.
28. Eat half my dinner portion and half my dessert, and save the leftovers for tomorrow.
29. Get rid of my microwave and all the processed food that goes in there.
30. Skip the middle aisles at the supermarket.
31. Make my food from scratch.
32. Grill, steam, or bake instead of frying my food.
33. Use vegetable oils instead of butter.
34. Eat less salt.
35. Increase the fiber in my diet.
36. Switch from white bread to whole grain bread.

37. Avoid refined white pasta.

38. Eat a whole lot more veggies of different colors.

39. Eat a piece of fruit every day.

40. Eat more fish.

41. Eat less red meat and more poultry.

42. Try new recipes that are free of gluten, refined sugar, dairy, and eggs.

Body Promises—I Will:

43. Stay away from the couch, which is a magnet for my butt.

44. Walk instead of drive whenever I can.

45. Get off the bus or subway one or two stops early and walk the rest of the way to my destination.

46. Park farther from the entrance at work and the store.

47. Take a brisk morning walk for energy.

48. Walk the kids to school.

49. Get up from my desk and walk around for five minutes every hour.

50. Take a walk during my breaks and lunch hour.

51. Take the family for a half-hour walk after dinner instead of watching TV.

52. Take the dog to the park every day.

53. Walk or run the dog around the park instead of standing still to play fetch.

54. Walk to work.

55. Ride my bike to and from work a few days a week.

56. Do my own housework instead of hiring it out.

57. Mow my lawn with a push mower.

58. Wash the car by hand.

59. Exercise for five minutes a day.

60. Work out in the morning before I do anything else.

61. Exercise during TV commercials.

62. Do fifteen push-ups, fifteen sit-ups, and fifteen squats every morning to start my day.

63. Choose cardio exercises that take me outdoors into the beautiful fresh air.

64. Join an exercise group or gym.

65. Take one new class or try one new piece of equipment at the gym this week.

66. Sign up for a community or charity walk/race.

67. Go to bed fifteen minutes earlier every night.

68. Sit up straight.

69. Stand instead of sitting whenever I can.

70. Smoke one less cigarette every day.

71. Take a multivitamin every day.

Mind Promises—I Will:

72. Look myself in the mirror every day and say, "I am worth it."

73. Breathe deeply.

74. Put on workout clothes the minute I get up each morning.

75. Make my bed and get dressed in street clothes every day.

76. Keep a checklist of the nonnegotiable things I *must* do every day.

77. Track and measure my eating and exercise, and write it down.

78. Keep my changes basic and reasonable.

79. Set small weekly goals instead of big, long-term goals.

80. Say "I will" instead of "I want" and "I can" instead of "I can't."

81. Act, instead of thinking about acting.

82. Count my day's accomplishments each night.

83. Reward myself for my accomplishments.

84. Forgive myself for one failure a day.

85. Find something good about myself every day, instead of something that's wrong with me.

86. Stop eating automatically while watching TV or using the computer.

87. Practice mindful eating—pay attention to what, when, where, how, and why.

88. Allow myself to say "no, thank you, I don't eat this."

89. Use food to nourish my body, not mask my emotions.

90. Stop eating my sadness.
91. Make a point of sitting down to family dinners to share the health.
92. Pay attention to the way I feel.
93. Share my feelings with others.
94. Give myself permission to cry.
95. List my emotional and food triggers and stay away from them.
96. Avoid negative and unhealthy people who bring me down.
97. Surround myself with like-minded people.
98. Get support.
99. Ask my friends to hold me accountable for my promises.
100. Take control of one decision each day and don't let anyone else make it for me.
101. Remind myself each day that "nobody will do it for me."

As you read through the Power Promises, a few of them probably jumped out at you and said "I'm the promise for you." These are the first promises you should make to yourself as you start your journey of transformation. Go back to the list and pick one to three promises from *each* category that you'd like to focus on first, no more. If you need to tweak a promise so it aligns better with your situation, don't hesitate to do so. Then write your promises down. Remember to choose promises you believe you can keep. Your integrity and dignity are on the line!

My Food Promises:

1.
2.
3.

My Body Promises:

1.
2.
3.

My Mind Promises:

1.
2.
3.

From among these, choose the very first promise you want to make to yourself. Make it something you can accomplish by the end of the day today. Put it down in writing.

Today, I promise myself I will:

Now, take a few steps that will help you fulfill your first promise, and many larger promises to come:

1. Write it down and post it in at least three places where you'll see it often.
2. Tell someone your promise and ask for that person's support. (You can also make it a status update on Facebook, a tweet on your Twitter account, and/or a declaration on my Facebook page!)
3. Identify the baby steps you need to take to meet this commitment to yourself. Take these steps one by one.
4. Identify the markers you can use to measure your progress toward fulfilling your promise.
5. Keep a daily log of your successes and setbacks.

At the end of the week, have you kept your promise? Did you eat every three hours? Take walks on your lunch break? Share your feelings with someone? If you did, give yourself a big pat on the back and a reward, such as that scarf you've had your eye on or that trip to the movies. If not, *don't be hard on yourself*. Work on your promise for as long as you need to.

Once you've kept your first Power Promise, choose another of the promises you wrote down above and focus on that for the next week. Keep going down the list—you're doing great!

The Third Secret: Fall Without Failing

Sometimes, even when we make small, attainable promises, or set small, attainable goals, we don't manage to keep them. What now? Are we destined to fail? Not at all. We only fail when we lose belief . . . give up . . . stop trying.

Look, nobody's perfect. We're all human, and life happens. We're all going to fall sometimes. In fact, we're going to fall many, many times in our lives! If you remember this—if you *expect to fall* once in a while—you won't be surprised when you do. You'll be prepared. I'm going to prepare you to fall without failing. See, there are three simple steps to getting back on your feet after you fall. Simple, but incredibly powerful.

If you're prepared with the knowledge of these three steps and are willing to follow them, you'll always be able to keep your falls from turning into failures. Take these steps whenever you stumble during your journey to transformation, and you *will* reach your goals! You'll be able to get back up after you fall if you confess, reassess, and recommit.

COURAGE TO CONFESS

The very first thing you need to do to recover from a fall is to confess. Get that emotional weight off your chest. Walk right over to a mirror, look yourself in the eye, and *confess to yourself* that you broke a promise you made to yourself or fell short of a goal. Don't keep any of the facts or feelings in. Let it all out! After you confess to yourself, *confess to somebody else.* Saying it out loud, to another person, makes your confession that much more powerful. Spell out the gory details, no matter how disgusting or embarrassing you think they are. Confession is one of the mightiest tools of transformation.

But I'll be honest with you: This is without a doubt the most difficult aspect of transformation. It sounds terrifying because you don't want to look bad in front of anybody else and risk scaring them off. Trust me, you won't. But you need to free yourself from shame and regret. It takes courage, authenticity, and determination. When you confess, to yourself and to another person, you take back *control of your life*. What you lost when you fell comes back to you.

REACH DOWN AND REASSESS

Once you own up to your mistakes, reassess the promises that you made to yourself. Why did you break them? Maybe something came up in your life that you used as an excuse to drop the ball. Maybe there was an unexpected life event and you spent the day stranded in an airport or emergency room. When you reassess a promise you broke for reasons like these, you can realistically expect to get right back on track tomorrow.

But maybe you bit off more than you could chew and set your goals too high. Maybe you're a single working mom with three kids who set herself the impractical goal to do two hours of cardio every day. Wow. That's one extreme promise! You'll definitely fall, so you need to reassess your expectations.

To keep falling from turning into failing, ask yourself sincerely if your vision is *realistic and attainable*. Is it really possible to reach those goals you set? Or do you need to reduce the weight of your commitment by aiming for more attainable targets? Remember, the carb-cycle program is totally adaptable to your needs and capabilities. If you *reassess and revise your goals*, you'll know that you can reach them, and you *will* reach them, and you'll believe in yourself again.

SMART Goals

What are your dreams for your body? Do you want to lose 20 pounds? 100 pounds? Do you want to get down to a cholesterol count of 180? A dress size of 10? To achieve transformation, your goals have to be crystal-clear. Without a detailed plan, your dreams have no direction—no purpose. *Goals* focus on hard-and-fast targets.

I help my clients put their weight-loss dreams into words using a proven technique called SMART goal-setting. Using this method, it's easy to map out and stay on your path to success. You can work out both short- and long-term goals.

The SMART system spells out the *five criteria* that a plan must meet in order to be effective.

SPECIFIC: Don't just say "I'm going to lose weight." This kind of vague, ambiguous promise makes it easy to bend the rules if you hit bumps in the road. Your commitment will crumble, and you'll destroy your self-respect. *Be explicit* when you lay out your plan: "I will work my way up to power-walking one mile" or "I will lose fifty-three pounds." Now you really know where you're headed!

MEASURABLE: Translate your plan into numbers, so you can measure *your progress toward your goal*. Numbers will keep you from kidding yourself about how you're doing! What's more, seeing your numbers move in the right direction will strengthen your motivation, while seeing them move in the wrong direction will refocus your efforts. Whether pounds, body measurements, clothing sizes, or health markers, choose one or two quantifiable transformation goals, such as how many inches you want to take off your waist or what you want your blood pressure to be. Track your numbers and use them to stay on course.

ATTAINABLE: Boost your chances of success by setting goals that you can actually attain. Line your goals up with the *realities* of your life: Do you have a heart condition? Do you work crazy hours? Do you hate fish? The carb-cycle program can flex with your situation, so make sure your goals take the facts into account. You have to move toward your goals every single day, so only set ones that are doable *for you*. Attainable goals make you feel great: Each time you reach one, you believe in yourself all over again.

RELEVANT: Does this goal have a significant meaning to you? Is it worth making it a priority in your life? To create a change in your body and health, you will need to create a change in your lifestyle. This can mean certain sacrifices must be made. Make sure that for you, the juice is worth the squeeze!

TIME-BOUND: Set a precise time frame for your transformation journey. For example, "I will reach my short-term goal by next Saturday. I will reach my long-term goal by my anniversary." Deadlines create a sense of urgency and keep you from procrastinating. They remind you that *your weight-loss commitments are important*. "Someday" and "eventually" weaken your resolve to reach your goals. Without the pressure of time to keep up your momentum, you'll grind to a halt and hate yourself for it. With the clock ticking, you'll run for the finish line!

Are your goals SMART? If they meet the SMART criteria, you're much more likely to reach them. Here are a few examples of SMART and not-so-SMART goals:

NOT-SO-SMART GOALS	SMART GOALS
Specific	
I want to get skinny.	I will wear a size six by my wedding date.
I'm going to exercise more.	I will work out three times a week for at least fifteen minutes at a time.
Measurable	
I'm going to drink less soda.	I will enjoy one diet soda each week.
I'll try to drink more water.	I will drink sixty-four ounces of water each day.
Attainable	
I want to be a yoga master.	I will take my first yoga class by July 31.
Relevant	
I will place top ten in the Boston Marathon next year.	I will lose seventy-five pounds in twelve months.
Time-Bound	
I'm going to cut back on junk food.	I will only eat junk food once a week, on my reward day.
I want to lose fifteen or twenty pounds.	I will lose fifteen pounds within three months. I will lose twenty pounds by December 15.

RISE UP AND RECOMMIT

Reassessing your transformation vision clarifies what's possible for you *right now*. You know what you can honestly promise yourself and what goals are SMART for you. You know that you can follow through when you take them on, and you believe in yourself again. You're not afraid of falling—you accept that you will—because you know you can get back up. Self-confidence empowers you to recommit to your weight-loss journey.

Toughen your commitment by *declaring your promises and goals*. Say them out loud. Write them down. Announce them to people that you love and trust. There's no more room for silent promises or ridiculous goals—the kind you can hide behind. Declaring your commitment makes it rock-solid. Now you can rev up your determination and get back on track with your transformation, knowing that in the future you will fall again, but not fail. Stride forward boldly!

The Fourth Secret: Unite

You've heard the expression,"No man [or woman!] is an island." Let me translate that: Humans need one another. We find strength in numbers, so we do everything together, as a group. That means you're not programmed or equipped to make your weight-loss journey alone. The support and encouragement of others help you believe in yourself and keep your promises to yourself. Your connections with other people create a safety net that lets you fall without failing. The *power* of your tribe *empowers* you: It's the wind at your back as you make your voyage to health and happiness!

It's been said that people become like their friends, loved ones, and associates (and even their pets!). If you want to be healthy, you should hang out with healthy people and absorb their energy. If you want to be happy, you should surround yourself with happy people. Interacting with those who are already where you want to be, learning from them and adopting their vision makes it easier to become who you want to be.

Group energy gives you a leg up on transformation in three big ways:

ACCOUNTABILITY

The first thing you must do after you put together your support network is *tell your people* what you're going to do and ask them to hold you to it. Most of the time, you make your diet promises in secret. I call them *silent promises*, because you don't declare them in front of anyone. You're so unsure of your willpower and fortitude that you're terrified to put your self-respect on the chopping block in front of others! When you break silent promises, you can sweep them under the rug. You don't have to answer to anyone.

It's way too easy to break a silent promise! That's why you need a support network. You're more likely to fulfill your weight-loss commitments to yourself if you share them with others—you don't want to let them down! When you make a mistake, *you can't let yourself off the hook* and repeat the vicious circle of more silent promises. So promise your people that you'll let them know when you stumble on your path to transformation.

To keep your weight-loss goals on track, you need to confess your slip-ups to your crew, which isn't easy. Sure—you already feel bad enough about botching up, and now your partners will hold you accountable for it. Confessing is scary and uncomfortable, and with your people wishing the best for you, you'll have to face the character-building challenge of getting back up—right in front of them! It just might be enough to keep you on the straight and narrow.

You want to make your team proud; you want them to believe in you. Let that desire to please them drive you until you have built the self-love and self-worth that can carry you along your journey. Once you reach your destination, you'll very likely find yourself expecting accountability from your team!

MOTIVATION

The praise and encouragement your tribe gives you are like rocket fuel for your transformation. When people on your team tell you how well they think you're doing, how good you look now that you're losing weight, you *want* to do more and go farther—not just for yourself, but for them. That's motivation. It feels good to believe in yourself and keep your promises, to reach your goals, and it can feel even better to make your cheer squad happy. Your drive and determination shoot through the roof! Your chances of weight-loss success go up exponentially.

HEALING

There's another upside of confessing to your partners: They'll make sure that when you fall, you don't fail. They'll lend you an understanding ear, help you reassess your goals and promises, and root for you as you recom-

How Do My Family and Friends Fit into the Picture?

You might not want to hear it, but I'll say it right up front: Your immediate family and friends may not be your best supporters. I strongly recommend that, right off the bat, you put every single member of your family on hold when it comes to your transformation team. This might disappoint you, but follow my advice on this. Granted, there are occasional exceptions out there, but in my experience, your husband or mother or sister may not belong on your team—it's just too emotionally complicated. The same might go for many of your friends: You must be completely, absolutely confident that they're on your side *100 percent*.

It's not that your family and friends are bad people, but their *vision* for you might not align with yours. Maybe you come from an overweight family that doesn't understand why you want to get in shape. Maybe your spouse is afraid that once you lose the weight you'll leave him. Maybe your best friend is a junk food junkie who'd feel rejected if you stopped scarfing nachos with her. That's all right! You love them, but these folks don't belong on your support squad, if this is the case. However, if they love and support your decision unconditionally, let their actions earn them a valuable spot on your team.

mit to yourself—and to them. When you reach out to your crew for encouragement in tough times, they'll be there for you. Tell them you're going to fall sometimes. Let them know that you'll be coming to them to heal and get back up on your feet. When they understand the steps of confessing, reassessing, and recommitting, they can and will hear your confessions warmly and compassionately. Their response will reinforce your courage to confess. Their love and faith—*their belief in you*—will help you heal. And as you heal, you can give back to them by persevering in your weight-loss journey. Their support makes it much, much easier to get back up and go forward.

PICKING YOUR TEAM

Putting together a winning team—one that can fully support you—is *essential* to your transformation success. These point people have the potential to make your journey a lot easier and more exhilarating. Once you identify some potential supporters, ask yourself four questions:

1. Do I trust them wholeheartedly?
2. Do I feel comfortable telling them anything?
3. Am I certain that they won't judge me or chew me out if I fall?
4. Can I confess to them again and again, knowing that they'll always thank me for my honesty?

So where do you find possible teammates? What kind of people should they be? Answer: people who already have what you want. It might seem difficult to find good point people. Possibly, there's no one you know who meets the criterion. Don't worry, it's *not a problem.* There are so many places to find open, compassionate people who share your journey. They might even need their own point people!

This questionnaire will get you thinking about who'd make the best TEAM YOU players.

My goal is:

....

....

What are the emotional, physical, and lifestyle characteristics of a person who has achieved this goal?

....

....

What do I need to change about myself or my life to become this person?

....

....

Who do I know who's achieved my goal? Who's currently pursuing my goal or one like it?

....

....

Does each of them have a positive attitude? Would each of them be a good cheerleader for me?

....
....

Who will I ask right now to be a member of my support team?

....
....

Where might I meet other people who have achieved or are currently pursuing my goal (gym, health food store, hobby, club, etc.)?

....
....

What websites or online communities might connect me with these like-minded people?

....
....

Which three places will I go to first to start meeting people who might belong on my support team?

    1.

    2.

    3.

Hey! Don't forget to include us on your support team! We might not be able to come to your house, but we've put together an app full of daily motivational tips and helps: Check out my website to find links to download it. And hit our social media sites to connect even more:

chrispowell.com
heidipowell.net
facebook.com/RealChrisPowell
facebook.com/HeidiPowell
twitter.com/RealChrisPowell
twitter.com/RealHeidiPowell

We'll be with you every step of the way on your transformation journey! We also recommend the following resources:

Weight Watchers (weightwatchers.com) offers meetings around the world as well as an online community. You can meet like-minded friends in either place.

Overeaters Anonymous (oa.org) is a twelve-step program that holds meetings all over the world. On their website you can find a meeting near you and get to know others who are transforming their lives.

FindSportsNow (findsportsnow.com) is an awesome source of info on sports groups, leagues, clubs, and athletic events in your community. Whether you're into walking, yoga, tennis, or weight training, this site connects you to people who share your goals.

3

WEIGHT LOSS 101

When Rachel was a little girl, she was sure that God had big plans for her, that He had something special in mind just for her. She knew she was a little different: She was the only one in her family with brown eyes, and she was the only one who struggled with weight problems. Growing up with four brothers and sisters, she'd come home from church and share a big, Southern family dinner, eating sometimes as much as 2,400 calories in one meal! Afterward, while clearing the table, she'd eat even more.

Rachel kept getting chunkier, so she had to stop doing some of the things she loved. She loved adrenaline rushes, but when she was thirteen she had to get off a ride at an amusement park because she didn't fit in the seat. Even though she was deeply embarrassed, she didn't let her feelings show. She fit in at school by being the smart, funny, outgoing kid. Despite her size, she was athletic, playing on the basketball team. Her only problem was her weight. By the time she was fifteen, Rachel weighed 315 pounds. Still, she didn't feel fat! When she looked in the mirror, she saw a beautiful young woman.

That began to change during Rachel's last year in high school. She realized that when some people looked at her, they didn't see a likeable, interesting girl; they saw a fat girl. She knew she needed to do something about her weight, but she had no clue where to begin. Assuming that if she ate less, she'd weigh less, she tried fad diet after fad diet. She just got tangled up in confusing numbers and calorie counting. After a week or two, she'd give up or move on to another plan. Nothing lasted.

Rachel went to college hoping she'd get her life back, but instead she kept eating the same unhealthy way she always had: one huge meal at a time. She starved herself during the day, then ate at night—two thousand or more calories all at once. The pattern seriously messed with her metabolism, which made it deadly for her weight. She had no clue about the damage she was doing to her body.

In three months, Rachel packed on eighty more pounds, reaching her highest weight—399 pounds. It was difficult for her to walk and even to breathe, let alone play the sports she loved. When she went home on break, her family was shocked. She started to give up on her dreams of achieving something great someday. She was completely miserable.

Health became a big problem for Rachel. Her doctor told her that she'd never be able to have children at her weight and ordered an ultrasound on her thyroid. When the doctor at the clinic asked her how much she weighed, she took a guess and said 350 pounds—too much for the clinic's table! Then Rachel heard about Lap-Band surgery and figured it was her key to success—to changing her life. But she didn't qualify for the operation. One setback after another took its toll.

Now what? Rachel decided that the NBC show *The Biggest Loser* was her ticket. When she was turned down, she tried to move on. She got a job teaching at a small Christian school, but she still couldn't control her eating and her weight remained a problem. As the gym teacher, she couldn't do half the exercises she taught the kids! She had always loved to play sports, and now she couldn't. Something in her mind clicked: Rachel wanted a good life, not one wasted on misery. If she was going to improve her life, she had to make some big changes. This was her moment of clarity—she just didn't know how to turn that clarity into action.

Then Rachel got a phone call about a new show, ABC's *Extreme Makeover: Weight Loss Edition*. She figured it wouldn't hurt to try out. So she wrote a letter to me and poured her heart out about how badly she wanted to transform her life, and promising to give my program her all. In tryouts she proved her determination. When I invited her onto the show, she was ecstatic. Little did she know that her life was about to change forever!

As we started working together, Rachel could feel the confidence I had in her—confidence that she didn't have in herself. For once in her life, she really believed she could drop hundreds of pounds, and she was ready to do whatever it was going to take. After some deep soul searching, she challenged herself to lose 50 percent of her body weight. It was a commitment to herself, but she also hoped she could become an inspiring example for other desperate people. This vision of her future was her motivation.

Before she met me, Rachel didn't know what a carb was. But now she learned all about the importance of carbs and the impact that nutrition has on her metabolism. She learned which foods could help her lose weight and which she should avoid. How to make balanced meals, how to control her portions, how to spread her meals out over the day: Rachel learned how to feed her body without hurting it.

One of the key elements of any successful long-term program was especially valuable for Rachel: the ability to cheat! Being able to splurge on her favorite foods helped her curb cravings, because she knew that if she couldn't have a cupcake or ice cream today, she could have it tomorrow. It was easier for her to stick with the program because to her, it didn't really feel like a diet.

Day by day, Rachel's confidence grew and she saw great results. After she lost her first one hundred pounds, medical tests showed she was perfectly healthy. Within a year, she lost 161 pounds! She hit some bumps in the road as she neared her goal weight—she couldn't afford groceries, so she ate with her family; her progress plateaued—but her expanding knowledge and self-esteem helped her conquer the problems.

Rachel's down to 208 pounds, and she's maintaining her weight. Carb-cycling has actually simplified her life! Nowadays she eats when she wakes up and then every two to three hours after that. She tries to drink a gallon of water daily. Her favorite low-carb foods are Ezekiel 4:9 brand breads and tortillas—they even make her feel like she's cheating! Sweet potatoes and baked potatoes are her favorite high-carb foods. As a binge-prone eater, she keeps things realistic by enjoying cheat meals three days a week.

It's a lifestyle that goes far beyond diet. Rachel's learned how to balance her work life with her social life and personal life. Plus, she's become a certifiable gym rat! She goes first thing every morning and whenever she wants to celebrate an accomplishment or blow off stress. When she's angry, she puts on her pink boxing gloves and hand wraps and beats the bag. The adrenaline junkie has reemerged, and she's trying all kinds of new things, like bungee jumping, that scare her. When faced with a challenge, she takes it on. And she loves meeting new people.

Rachel feels like she took a lump of dirt and created a masterpiece. Her story is an amazing example of what a healthy diet and a little exercise can do for you: It can change your life! Success like Rachel's is within your reach. Before she started carb-cycling, Rachel was scared and overwhelmed—she didn't think it was possible to transform her life. But in her moment of clarity she decided that she was worth the extra effort, the hard work, to give herself a happier, healthier life. When you open them up, the human mind and

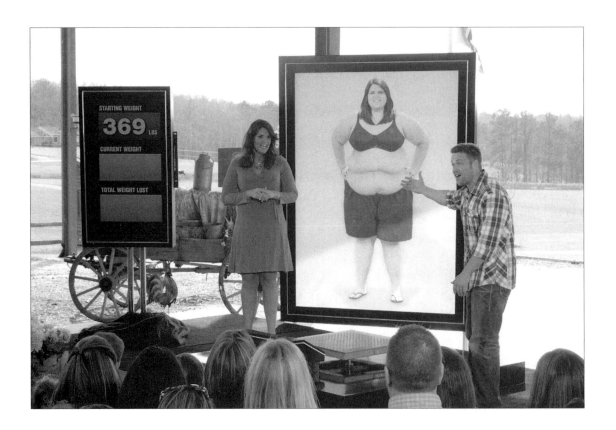

human heart are amazing things! That's exactly what Rachel did, and because she did she's proven that anything is possible.

The moment of clarity, when it happens, is different for everyone. For some it may be when they hit a brutal rock bottom, for others it may simply emerge from curiosity about what a better future might look like. When you have yours, the desire for a new lifestyle will spark to life within you. Your desire will grow and grow, finally bursting forth as motivation. That's what will turn your clarity and desire into action. That's when you're ready to get going with carb cycling. That's what will make your transformation journey a fantastic success!

Changing It Up

So what's the big deal about carb cycling? In a nutshell, it's a way of eating that *alternates days of high-carbohydrate meals with days of low-carbohydrate meals*—and allows you to reward yourself regularly along the way! Carbohydrates come from plants and are the major component of foods like bread, potatoes, pasta, corn, beans, fruits, vegetables, and sugar-heavy "bad carbs" such as soda and candy. Carbs have certainly gotten a bad rap over the last couple decades, but there are profound benefits to eating good carbs! They're the fuel source that your muscles and organs prefer.

Carbs fire up your body's calorie-burning metabolic furnace, and you can *make the most of that process* by carb-cycling. On days when you eat more carbs, you stoke the furnace, and on days when you eat fewer carbs, your furnace burns fat like crazy. The high-carb/low-carb pattern tricks your metabolism into burning hot even on days when it doesn't get many carbs, so it starts ripping through body fat. That's one way carb-cycling maximizes weight loss!

I've developed a carb-cycling program that's doable for nearly everyone and consistent at getting amazing results. It will help you achieve your weight-loss and fitness goals incredibly quickly without requiring a huge amount of effort. You can use this approach to drop as many pounds as you wish, and when you stick with it, you'll be able to maintain your ideal weight and stay in excellent shape *for the rest of your life*!

Before we get into the nitty-gritty of my system, here's a little background info that'll help you understand your weight and make it easier for you to get hold of the carb-cycling process.

Burn Baby Burn

If you're out to shrink your waistline (and any other measurement!), you want to burn fat as fast as you safely can. In order to prime your body to start losing weight and keep on losing weight, you've got to follow three rules. They may surprise you:

Rule 1: Eat more carbs and eat more often.
Rule 2: Develop shapely muscles.
Rule 3: Move your muscles.

Are you kidding me, Chris? More meals, more carbs, and more muscle—that can't make me skinnier! But in fact, feeding your body *in the right way*, together with growing and shaping your muscles, will power up your metabolism—and keep it powered up—so it blazes right through your fat. It's textbook physiology! I'll lay it all out for you a little later in this chapter.

The Three Fires

First, let's make sure you understand how your metabolism works. I covered the details in my first book, *Choose to Lose*, so you probably already know that the term *metabolism* refers to the way your body uses energy to power your organs and muscles. That energy is measured in units called calories. Where does all that energy go? Your metabolism burns calories for three purposes:

- *Digestion:* You probably don't realize it, but your body burns calories when it digests and absorbs the food you eat. Around 10 to 15 percent of the calories you use every day gets eaten up here. The *quantity and quality* of those calories lay the hormonal foundation of weight loss.

- *Being (Resting Metabolic Rate):* The calories that don't get burned up during digestion get used by your organs: your beating heart, your breathing diaphragm, your filtering liver, and all the others. When you're not moving, your *resting muscles* use calories as they repair and remodel themselves. The basic functioning of your body accounts for 60 to 75 percent of the calories you burn daily.

- *Movement:* When you move, putting your muscles to work, they need a lot of fuel—20 to 35 percent of the calories you use. That's just for *ordinary motion*: Endurance athletes burn up to 50 percent of their calories to power their muscles!

YOUR METABOLISM
How You Burn Calories Every Day

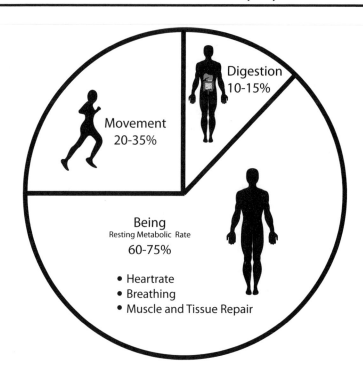

That's the *how* of calorie-burning; now here's the *how much*. The number of calories you burn each day varies according to how active you are. If you follow the same routine every day, eating and moving around (or not) in pretty much the same ways, you'll burn roughly the same number of calories every day. The proportion of calories used by each of your body's three energy users—digestion, being (resting metabolic rate), and movement—will also stay pretty constant.

So how many calories are we talking about? That depends on four things: your age, your weight, your height, and your gender. All other things being equal, a bigger body needs more calories than a smaller one does, and a younger body needs more calories than an older body does. Take a look at the chart on the opposite page to see your estimated baseline calorie usage. It shows how many calories a body your size and age typically burns in a day with light movement.

Figuring Out Your Figure

All these numbers are swell, but you're reading this book because you want to slim down, not because you want to study science. Let's put the facts and figures together into tools that will help you get the body you want. The arithmetic of weight loss is super-simple:

- Each day that you eat more calories than your metabolism burns, your body stores the extra energy as body fat. You gain weight.
- Eat the same number of calories as your metabolism burns, and your body neither builds nor uses up its stores of fat. You maintain your weight.
- Eat fewer calories than your metabolism burns, and your body makes up the energy shortfall by tapping into your fat. You lose weight. This is what fitness professionals call a *calorie deficit*, and it's the key to weight loss.

The calorie deficit is what weight loss is all about. If you want to drop the pounds, you have to run your metabolism at a deficit. How big a deficit?

ESTIMATED CALORIE EXPENDITURE
(Calories Burned Daily)

Average Man, 5'8" Tall

Age→	20 Years	30 Years	40 Years	50 Years	60 Years	70 Years	80 Years
Weight (lbs.)↓							
125-150	2318	2230	2142	2054	1966	1878	1790
150-175	2521	2433	2345	2257	2169	2081	1993
175-200	2724	2636	2548	2460	2372	2284	2196
200-250	3130	3042	2954	2866	2778	2690	2602
250-300	3334	3246	3157	3069	2981	2893	2805
300-350	3740	3652	3564	3476	3388	3299	3211
350-400	4146	4058	3970	3882	3794	3706	3618
400-500	4755	4667	4579	4491	4403	4315	4227

Average Woman, 5'4" Tall

Age→	20 Years	30 Years	40 Years	50 Years	60 Years	70 Years	80 Years
Weight (lbs.)↓							
100-125	1827	1766	1705	1645	1584	1523	1462
125-150	1968	1907	1847	1786	1725	1664	1603
150-175	2109	2049	1988	1927	1866	1805	1745
175-200	2251	2190	2129	2068	2008	1947	1886
200-250	2533	2472	2412	2351	2290	2229	2168
250-300	2674	2614	2553	2492	2431	2371	2310
300-350	2957	2896	2835	2775	2714	2653	2592
350-400	3240	3179	3118	3057	2996	2936	2875
400-500	3663	3603	3542	3481	3420	3359	3299

Here's the magic number: To lose one pound of fat in a given window of time—say, a week—you've got to burn 3,500 more calories than you take in. That doesn't mean you have to cut out 3,500 calories a day (you probably don't even eat that much!). But to lose weight you do have to eat less. Most carb-cyclers find that they get the best results by creating a 500- to 1,000-calorie deficit daily.

The good part about all this math is that you're not stuck with the "average" metabolism that burns the "typical" number of calories listed in the metabolic rate chart. *You can get a bigger calorie deficit* by making your metabolism burn hotter, so it incinerates calories like there's no tomorrow. By manipulating your metabolism, you can burn more calories than the imaginary people in that chart! How do you do that? By carb cycling, of course! Cycling your carbs creates a calorie deficit that *guarantees fat loss.* Now let's get back to those three crazy rules for maximizing your metabolism.

Uncommon Sense

Like I said a few pages back, there are three rules for burning fat and losing weight quickly. I might sound crazy, but I promise that if you follow these rules, you'll get the body you want—faster than you thought you could. But you've got to stick with all three of them, and here's why:

RULE 1: EAT MORE CARBS AND EAT MORE OFTEN.

Eating more stimulates your body's digestion and maintenance functions. Your metabolism rises and falls with your calorie intake and fires in three-hour cycles. If it's got a lot of fuel at the right time, it burns at its hottest. This is why you should eat more often—every three hours, to be exact—for a total of five meals a day. Of course, you have to eat the right kind of food, namely carbs, your body's favorite fuel. If you don't throw enough fuel on the fire, the flames fizzle out. Just as a log that you toss on a pile of ashes just sits there, calories that you feed to a sluggish metabolism just sit there and get stored in the form of fat.

Carbs are the major macronutrient in plant-based foods like sweet potatoes, oatmeal, beans, and fruit. (They're also the main component of not-so-healthy stuff like hamburger buns, soda, and glazed donuts, but not all carbs deserve a bad rap.) Carbs are, first and foremost, the main food for your cells. But they're also the switch that calibrates your body's metabolic thermostat, playing a significant role in controlling how fast your metabolism burns calories. When carbs come your way, they stimulate your body to release special hormones that are essential in managing your metabolism. Eating more carbs sends more of these hormones into your system, and the hormones launch your metabolic rate sky-high. Eating fewer carbs slows the flow of hormones, suppressing your metabolism. Carbs set your metabolic thermostat to "hot." The trick is eating the right amount of them, at the right time, and we'll get to that in a bit. Moral of the story: Eat more carbs and eat them more often!

RULE 2: DEVELOP SHAPELY MUSCLES.

If you develop your muscles, your body's maintenance and movement functions get stronger. Pumping up your muscles with weights or other resistance techniques actually breaks them down, so for the next twenty-four to forty-eight hours, your body hammers overtime to repair and remodel them. This takes a *ton* of energy, so guess what? Your metabolism goes through the roof while your body builds shapelier and stronger muscles than ever! Plus, moving your muscles at high intensity for short periods of time creates a metabolic afterburn that lasts for hours after you exercise. If you work out regularly, your body becomes a fat-burning furnace—even when you're flopped on the couch watching TV. Moral of the story: Shape up your muscles.

RULE 3: MOVE YOUR MUSCLES.

Moving your muscles improves your body's movement function. Put them in motion, and we're talking metabolic explosion. When you move your body, your muscles quickly start devouring calories. Your muscle cells scarf down way more energy than any other cells in your body, so when you make them work, your metabolism cranks up to white-hot.

The more muscle you have, the more calories it eats, and when your metabolism is burning high to feed your muscles, *all* of your cells—not just your muscle cells—end up using more calories, even while you're sleeping! Moral of the story: Move your muscles!

Why Cycle Carbs?

By following the three rules, you maximize your metabolism so you can create the calorie deficit you need to strip away your body fat. So where does carb cycling fit in? Simple: It takes your metabolism even farther up into the stratosphere!

Cycling your carbs—eating a lot every other day and very few on the days in between—is so effective at intensifying weight loss while maintaining fat-burning muscle that most bodybuilders and fitness models have been carb cycling for decades. Using this method with many of my clients over the years, I've taken what I've learned from their experiences and have developed my own system. It not only supercharges weight loss for all kinds of folks, it also fits into almost anyone's hectic everyday life. Plus, I've built in one to three days a week when you get to reward yourself with the decadent foods you love. And sometimes you get to eat tons of carbs for *a whole week*!

Of course, you can drop pounds on any diet that creates a calorie deficit, when you take in fewer calories than you use up. But many weight-loss regimens leave you feeling deprived by banning a lot of foods—most often, the delicious ones. Some diets, especially low-carb ones, actually *crash* your metabolism, slowing it way down and actually decelerating weight loss. Diet deprivation and metabolic crashing often lead to *rebounding* after you finish a diet, when you regain the weight you lost. Even more troubling, eliminating carbs from your diet can cause long-term damage to your hormonal system.

Carb cycling heads off the problems caused by other kinds of diets, but it still lets you lose weight rapidly. And unlike so many other weight-loss plans, carb cycling is effective in both the short and long term! By carb cycling—eating a lot of *beneficial* carbs on alternating days—you can set your metabolism to "high" on high-carb days and keep it from slowing down too much on low-carb days. Alongside high-quality carbs, you'll eat the valuable vegetables, proteins, and good fats that will enhance the benefits of carb cycling to maximize both fat loss and muscle development.

My carb-cycling program gets another boost from a technique that I call *calorie cycling*. Basically, you eat more calories on your high-carb days and fewer on your low-carb days. Why? Because your body burns calories, not carbs! Carbs *contain* the calories that fuel your body. When a lot of calories—whether fat, protein, or carb—come in, your metabolism quickly rises to turn them into lots of energy for your cells. When fewer calories come in, it slowly begins to fall, trying to eventually preserve as much energy as it can. That's why I've designed my carb cycles to increase your calorie intake on high-carb days and decrease it on low-carb days. More carbs + more calories = metabolic boost and fat burning; fewer carbs + fewer calories = slow metabolic drop and faster fat burning. Cycling calories along with carbs maximizes their combined impact on your metabolism. It prolongs the metabolic boost you get on high-carb days to create the largest calorie deficit possible on low-carb days. It's successful metabolic manipulation—the ultimate one-two punch for fat loss!

How to Work It

By now you know that carb cycling consists of alternating high-carb and low-carb eating days. Cycling carbs keeps your metabolism—your body's inner furnace—stoked to its hottest every hour of every day, even on low-carb days when you're not feeding it much fuel. There are a lot of ways to modify the pattern and the details to meet your specific needs, but the basic method—my Classic Carb Cycle—is a great place to begin.

The Classic Carb Cycle
Sunday—Free Day/High-Carb Day
Monday—Low-Carb Day
Tuesday—High-Carb Day

Wednesday—Low-Carb Day
Thursday—High-Carb Day
Friday—Low-Carb Day
Saturday—High-Carb Day and Weekly Weigh-In

When to Eat: Each day, whether it's a high-carb, low-carb, or reward day, eat five meals, no more and no less. Start your day at about the same time every day (any time is fine, as long as it's consistent) and *eat within 30 minutes of getting up* to crank up your metabolic furnace for the day. Then eat another meal every three hours for a total of five meals in the day. It's *essential* to time your meals on this schedule to keep your metabolism blazing away at its hottest and using up what you eat when you eat it.

Eating at three-hour intervals fuels your inner furnace to burn superhot between meals, melting your body fat. If you go longer than three hours without food, your furnace cools down. The calories you take in won't go up in flames. They'll just sit there until your body turns them into more fat! What if you're not hungry and don't feel like eating every three hours? *Eat anyway—no matter what.*

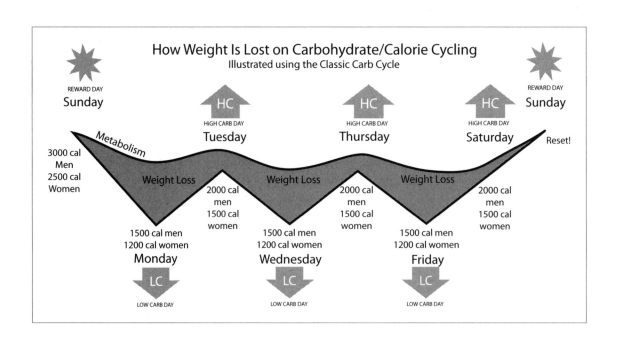

What to Expect: Five Meals a Day?!

Anytime you try to change your body's habitual patterns, your body will resist and for a while you'll feel uncomfortable—or downright lousy. Every organ in your body, from your brain and your adrenal glands to your stomach and your pancreas, will have to get used to your new ways, and until each of them does, you might not be happy about the changes! So don't be worried if switching over to the carb-cycle meal schedule feels awkward at first: *It's only natural.*

When you start eating five meals a day, what you'll notice most is that you will probably feel too full. Real, whole foods like the ones on this program tend to have a lot of volume, not a lot of calories! Three hours between meals won't seem like enough, and you won't always want to eat every meal. I know, it'll probably always sound weird, but to lose weight *you must eat a lot.* You have no choice: You've *got* to eat all five meals, every day!

Power through your body's resistance to eating so much, and don't worry . . . in *about three days* things will settle down. You will set new patterns for your body, and your inner furnace will be roaring away, tearing through everything you toss into it. You'll have more energy and feel better than ever, and you'll be hungry every three hours. Now, start eating and crank up that metabolic furnace!

Here's an example of a carb-cycling meal schedule, with a 6:45 A.M. wake-up time:

7:00 A.M.—breakfast

10:00 A.M.—morning snack

1:00 P.M.—lunch

4:00 P.M.—afternoon snack

7:00 P.M.—dinner

Keep in mind that this is just an example. Whether you're an early riser or work the midnight shift, you should always eat your first meal within thrity minutes of waking, and then eat every three hours after!

What to Eat: Okay, so what kind of food will you be eating all day? We're not talking about high-carb french fries and low-carb sausage! To keep your metabolism at peak efficiency and your body at peak performance, you have to feed yourself *the right fuel.* In Chapter 6, "Feed Your Fire: The Recipes," I'll give you a big list of the best foods for carb cycling.

Proteins: Grilled steak, roasted chicken, broiled fish, Greek yogurt—your taste buds and your body love protein. I'm going to ask you to *eat lean protein at every one of your five daily meals.* It builds and maintains energy-hungry muscle that burns calories like an inferno. It accelerates your overall metabolism to demolish even more calories. What's more, protein breaks down more slowly than carbs and fat, using up even more calories and keeping you fuller longer. When you eat protein, you also digest other nutrients more slowly, sustaining your energy level longer. Aside from lean meat, poultry, and fish, great sources of low-fat protein are cottage cheese, nonfat plain Greek yogurt, soy products such as tofu, and whey protein (for mixing into smoothies—yum!). All of these also contain lots of other good stuff that your body loves. Protein is the cornerstone of carb cycling and the centerpiece of all your meals.

Carbohydrates: Carbs are the main nutrient in foods that come from plants. Sounds healthy, right? Well, sometimes, sometimes not: There are junk and processed carbs, and then there are real carbs. It may come from corn, or beets, or sugarcane, but the sugar in candy bars is far from good for you. It's a *simple* carbohydrate, which means it breaks down superfast in your body and moves rapidly from your bloodstream to your muscle and fat cells. It sounds backward, but by eating sugar you end up with low blood sugar! When you eat processed carbs, like white flour and sugar, your blood sugar surges to dangerously high levels, triggering a hormonal reaction that ultimately leads to a devastating blood-sugar crash. That translates into low energy and a slowed metabolism. Good carb sources, though—sweet potatoes, berries, black beans, pears, peas, oatmeal, and many more—do your body a slew of favors. These are *complex* carbs, which break down slowly, keep your blood sugar steady, maximize long-

What to Expect: Killing Your Cravings

When your body's at a calorie deficit and burning fat, visions of pizza . . . potato chips . . . ice cream . . . all your no-no comfort foods will probably dance in your head. You can do a few things to keep yourself from sliding down the sugary, fatty slope:

- Start your day with a *high-fiber* breakfast (which will keep you from overeating later).
- Fill up with *water* throughout the day and avoid dehydration (which is proven to trigger cravings).
- Put something *minty*—sugar-free breath mints or gum, even tooth-paste—in your mouth (the flavor suppresses appetite).
- If an incredibly strong craving pops up on a low-carb day, eat just a little portion of *healthy fat* and drink some water. Within fifteen to twenty minutes, your craving should be under control!

lasting energy, and keep your inner furnace hot, hot, hot! The short version of the carb story is: complex carbs = a vigorous metabolism. They're the powerful variable of carb cycling.

Vegetables: Vegetables fall into the carbohydrates category, but since they're mostly low-carb and they're a huge part of carb cycling, I put them into their own group. Veggies are hugely nutritious and send all kinds of good stuff to every part of your body. Everything from your heart to your immune system benefits from a veggie-filled diet, and the antioxidants in veggies help prevent cancer! You can eat as many of these low-calorie beauties as you like, and since they come in such a variety of tasty flavors, shapes, and textures—green beans, spinach, carrots, onions, and so many others—*you won't get bored*. Filled with fiber, veggies keep you feeling full for a good, long time. Without a doubt, veggies are the perfect food when you're out to get rid of your fat.

Healthy Fat: Speaking of fat, I'll let you in on a delicious fact: *You can eat fat* when you're carb cycling! Healthy fat, that is. We're talking about peanut butter, string cheese, eggs, and a whole assortment of other plant- and dairy-based foods. When you're carb cycling, you can eat healthy fat on your low-carb days. You're already getting enough calories on your high-carb days, so you should stay away from fat then. But on low-carb days, a little healthy fat will keep your energy from dipping too low, and will keep you from feeling too hungry. Don't eat too much, though, or this high-calorie stuff will hold back your weight-loss mission.

How to Eat: When you're carb cycling, it's vital to put together the "when to eat" and "what to eat" components the right way to get the best, fastest possible results. Here's how to do it:

ON HIGH-CARB DAYS: BOOST YOUR METABOLISM		
When to Eat	What to Eat	What Happens
breakfast within 30 minutes of waking up	protein + carb + veggies	wakes up your metabolism and gives your body the fuel it needs to start the day
every 3 hours until you reach 5 meals	protein + carb + veggies	jacks up your metabolism, fuels your organs and muscles, and delivers vitamins and fiber

ON LOW-CARB DAYS: BURN THE FAT		
When to Eat	What to Eat	Results
breakfast within 30 minutes of waking up	protein + carb + veggies	wakes up your metabolism and gives your body the fuel it needs to start the day
every 3 hours until you reach 5 meals	protein + fat + veggies	burns fat, maintains your muscles, balances your hormones, and delivers vitamins and fiber

ON REWARD DAYS: RESET YOUR SYSTEM		
When to Eat	What to Eat	Results
breakfast within 30 minutes of waking up	Enjoy your reward foods in moderation! (see Appendix C, "Reward Foods," at the end of the book)	satisfies your cravings, rewards you for your progress, increases your calorie intake to maintenance level, and maintains your muscles
every 3 hours until you reach 5 meals	Enjoy your reward foods in moderation!	jacks up your metabolism and develops your calorie-burning muscles.

How to Keep It Going: Every once in a while, it's a good idea to restart your carb-cycling engine. Even though the high-carb/low-carb pattern prevents your body from adapting to a predictable intake of calories every day, which keeps your metabolism hot even when it should be cool, your intelligent body will eventually wise up to your tricks. When that happens, your metabolism will drop off and your weight loss will slow down or even stop. To restart the process, you've got to change up the way you're eating yet again.

Once a month you'll devote a week to the Slingshot Technique. During this week, every day will be a high-carb day. Eat exactly as you do on normal high-carb days, and by the seventh day your metabolism will be blazing away again. When you go back to carb cycling, your body will forget the trick you pulled on it before and start losing weight again. What's more, the Slingshot Technique gives your body extra rest and nourishment that allow it to recover from three weeks of carb cycling.

Capitalize on Exercise

Any successful weight-loss plan includes exercise as a central component, and my carb-cycling program is no exception. I've designed two types of quick workouts to *accelerate your weight loss*: muscle-building and cardiovascular. They go with carb cycling perfectly because they compound its

What to Expect:
Things to Look Out For

So you're carb cycling away, eating the right foods at the right times. How do you know you're getting anywhere? You do a weekly weigh-in each Saturday (no more often than that, as your weight fluctuates from day to day!), but sometimes from week to week *you might not see a change in that number on the scale.* Don't worry about it—it doesn't mean you're not making progress! In fact, you're most likely burning fat as your body develops new muscle—which burns fat faster. There are other, more reliable, signs to show that your body is responding exactly the way it should:

- The fit of your clothes (they should be getting looser; this is the very best indicator of where you're at)
- Your physical and mental energy level (you'll notice extra energy on high-carb days)
- Your appetite and craving levels (just a heads-up: cravings *might* be higher on low-carb days)
- Water retention (you should be peeing more on low-carb days than on high-carb days)
- Sleep quality (you might fall asleep faster after a high-carb day, but you should feel better rested after a low-carb day due to the increased output of growth hormone)

effects! Every weekday morning you do special muscle-building workouts. I call them 9-Minute Missions because in only nine minutes they move your metabolism-boosting mission forward. To accelerate your fat loss, do your customized cardio exercises anytime after your 9-Minute Missions. I call them Shredders because they tear through fat like nobody's business. Chapter 5, "Shape Your Body, Shred Your Fat: The Exercises" shows you everything you need to know; this is just a preview.

9-Minute Missions to Shape Your Muscles: Muscle-shaping exercise, also known as resistance training, heats up your metabolism by increasing the size of your energy-hungry muscles—the number one calorie users in your body. (It also shapes up your muscles so your body takes on its most attractive contours as you lose weight.) I've streamlined basic resistance training into 9-Minute Missions that can easily fit into your day.

When you're carb cycling, the 9-Minute Missions make the biggest impact if you do them first thing in the morning—before you eat breakfast—because they prime your metabolism to run at its peak for the rest of the day. I like to roll out of bed, do my Mission, and step right into the shower before sitting down to eat. However, if your schedule will not accommodate training first thing in the morning, any time of day will still give you phenomenal results.

Keeping it simple and natural, I've built the 9-Minute Missions around some of the human body's most basic movements: running, jumping, pushing, pulling, crunching, and squatting. Every exercise in these workouts uses a movement that your body is naturally designed to do. All of these movements are truly functional: They're downright *necessary* for human mobility and survival!

Since it's engineered to run, jump, push, pull, crunch, and squat, your body responds fastest to exercise based on these movements, as opposed to exercises that force it into movements it's not intended to do. This means you get better results with less effort than you would on some of that insane equipment at the gym or fitness studio. Which reminds me: You can do your 9-Minute Missions at home, without any expensive, space-hogging gear.

In Chapter 5, "Shape Your Body, Shred Your Fat," I introduce you to thirty muscle-shaping exercises that we use to create our 9-Minute Missions. Being able to switch between exercises from day to day keeps working out *fun*—not to mention extremely productive. Each of the Shaper Missions includes three of the muscle-building exercises that I've designed.

Those are the basics of building muscle while carb cycling. The best basic of all might be that the 9-Minute Missions take only . . . well, *nine minutes*. Nine minutes, five times a week! What an awesome way to get fit! What an easy way to charge up your metabolism!

Cardio Shredders to Strip Off Pounds: Although it's less intense than resistance training, cardio exercise is the optimum fat burner. Getting your muscles moving and your heart pumping will take your metabolism through the roof, and *your fat will melt right off.* When it comes to weight loss, this is what Shredders are all about. But they also deliver tons of oxygen to your organs, make your heart stronger, and do a bunch of other great things for your health!

When you think of cardio exercise, you might envision people sweating on elliptical machines or jumping around in aerobics class, but ordinary exercises, like swimming, biking, and walking, are just as good at working your cardiovascular system and burning fat. The key is to find an activity you love: gym classes, hiking, skating—you choose. You're a lot more likely to do your Shredders if you're having fun! They'll be even more fun—not to mention better at chomping calories—if you switch between different kinds of exercise once in a while.

When you're carb cycling, you do Shredders every day of the week except on the weekend. Each Shredder takes you through *two levels* of your chosen exercise: low-intensity and high-intensity. This might translate, for instance, to intervals of walking and then jogging. The shredders start out at five minutes in duration and increase five more minutes every week until you reach sixty minutes

For carb cyclers of average fitness, I recommend starting by "shredding" your existing cardio routine. What I mean is simply create intervals with whatever you are already doing and keep the duration the same. Then increase five minutes every week until you reach sixty minutes. Remember, the more Shredders you do, the more fat you burn!

Your Workout Week: With all these exercises and types of workouts, you might be a little confused about when to do which workout. No need to stress: In its basic form, the carb-cycling exercise schedule is actually straightforward and is laid out in easy-to-read charts throughout the book.

Some Very Large Carrots

Eating right and exercising—that's not all there is to weight loss, and certainly not all there is to transforming your life. But by changing what you eat and how you exercise throughout the week, by eating at the right time of day, and by coordinating your workouts with your diet, you can lose all the weight you want to, and keep trim and fit *for life*. Carb cycling makes weight loss as fast and easy as it can be, and you don't even have to give up the foods you love. That's a whole lot of carrots—without the stick. That's carb cycling!

Keep reading, and you'll find out that carb cycling is the best way to transform your life through weight loss because:

- It gives you the tools to control your metabolism so you can lose weight and body fat.
- It is totally customizable to your life and lifestyle.
- It allows you to eat the foods you crave and still lose weight.
- It conquers the dieter's plateau.
- It enables you to build lean, strong muscles.
- It helps you increase your energy level and overall health.
- It gives you a whole new understanding of and appreciation for your body.
- It hands you control of your body and your weight for the rest of your life.
- It empowers you physically, mentally, emotionally, and socially.

Let's do this!

4

WHAT'S YOUR CARB CYCLE?
FOUR PLANS FOR RAPID WEIGHT LOSS

Carb cycling really worked for Michael: He lost sixty-two pounds in three months! The key to his success, and his advice to other carb cyclers? *Don't quit.* No big mystery, right?

Michael started gaining weight when he left the navy. As a serviceman he'd been a trim 200 pounds, but as a civilian he blew up to 252. Working all the time, he *didn't pay attention* to what he was eating or how much he ate, and he didn't exercise at all. But even though he knew his lifestyle was unhealthy, he never expected to get so big! When he did, it hit his self-image—hard. He had a tough time climbing the stairs, and he'd get winded when he played with his son. This was not the Michael he knew. This was not the Michael he wanted to be.

It took some time and some soul-searching before Michael decided to do something about his weight. He'd never tried to slim down—he had picky eating habits and thought that going on a diet meant he'd have to eat foods he didn't enjoy. But he started thinking about the "before," where he was, 252 pounds, and the "after," where he wanted to be, back down to 200 pounds. He wasn't sure he could do it, but his wife gave him tons of encouragement to go for it. She believed in him and knew he could lose the weight.

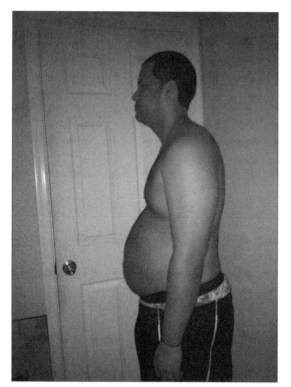

Then Michael discovered carb cycling and found out he could eat all kinds of foods and still lose weight. Holy cow! He could still *eat his favorite foods*—even pizza, his biggest weakness—on cheat days. "This looks pretty painless," he thought. "I can handle it!" He started out making small commitments to himself—preparing his food in advance, including lots of different veggies—and found that he could keep them! He got so confident that he decided right off the bat to do the Turbo Cycle, which is pretty demanding but would get him to his goal faster.

Every morning when he got up, Michael broke down his carb-cycle menu for the day. He kept his meal plans really *simple* but made sure they *weren't boring*, by including a lot of different foods that he liked. He stayed on top of his portion sizes and drank lots of water so he'd feel full between meals. Soon, Michael found that he was able to stick with carb cycling without feeling deprived, and his body and mind began to feel better.

But Michael faced challenges, too. His wife wasn't eating the same food on the same schedule, so it was difficult to sit down and share a meal together. But *he didn't quit*. Michael's wife kept cheering him on, and he lost thirty pounds in thirty days! His commitment skyrocketed.

One at a time, Michael continued to make small transformation promises to himself, and consistently kept them. His journey got easier as he started seeing results, and his belief in himself got stronger and stronger. Even after those first thirty days, when his progress slowed down, he hung in there. He was able to *break through his plateau* by using the slingshot technique, and dropped right back into the turbo cycle. Finally, after three months of carb cycling, Michael not only hit his target weight, but lost an extra ten pounds to boot. He didn't want junk food anymore—in fact, it made him feel sick—and he was bursting with energy. Michael was back!

You're committed to carb cycling. You've pledged to lose weight. You've resolved to transform your life. You're dedicated to keeping your promises to yourself. But it can be hard to be faithful to *you*, so start out by making little contracts with yourself. Fulfilling each tiny commitment—even just one—is a victory that will make you stronger. With each small victory, you'll be able to keep more and more and bigger and bigger promises to yourself. Your self-confidence and self-belief will grow and grow, and before you know it, you'll transform your life!

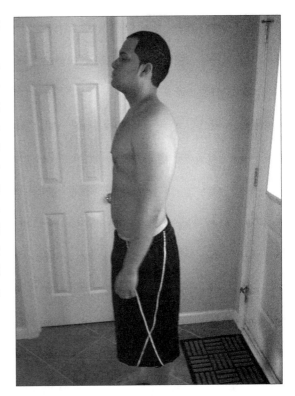

Cycling Is Simple

The beauty of carb cycling is that all you really have to remember is how to *eat in two different ways*. On some days—your high-carb days—you eat a lot of carbohydrates, and on the others—your low-carb days—you don't. You eat smart fats instead. It's that simple. Just put these two kinds of days together into a seven-day pattern that you follow from week to week, and you're carb cycling! It's amazing that the high-carb/low-carb cycle, such a straightforward setup, is such a powerful strategy for weight loss.

On *low-carb days*, you start out each and every day with a breakfast that includes a portion of protein, a portion of carbs, and as many vegetables as you want. You eat this within half an hour of getting up. After that, every three hours you eat a meal of one portion of protein, a portion of veggies, and one portion of fat. That's right, *fat*. Your total is *five meals a day*, with just enough carbs first thing in the morning to jump-start the metabolism. Pretty clear-cut. That's a low-carb day.

On *high-carb days*, you eat the same metabolic boosting breakfast that you do on low-carb days, within thirty minutes of waking up. Then you do things a little differently. Every three hours, for four more meals—for a total of five meals in the day—you have a meal made up of a portion of protein, a portion of carbs, and a portion of veggies. Easy, right? That's a high-carb day.

Now you're asking how much food's in a portion. Depends on what kind

CARB CYCLING DAYS
for EASY | CLASSIC | TURBO | FIT cycles

	Low Carb Day	High Carb Day	
BREAKFAST (within 30 minutes of waking)	PROTEIN + CARB	PROTEIN + CARB	
MORNING SNACK	PROTEIN + FAT	PROTEIN + CARB	**MEALS** (Eat every 3 hours and include 2 handfuls of veggies with each meal)
LUNCH	PROTEIN + FAT	PROTEIN + CARB	VEGETABLES
AFTERNOON SNACK	PROTEIN + FAT	PROTEIN + CARB	
DINNER	PROTEIN + FAT	PROTEIN + CARB	

ESTIMATED CALORIE INTAKE GOALS:	WOMEN	1,200	1,500
	MEN	1,500	2,000

SMART PROTEINS
Protein is essential for weight loss since it helps build muscle. The recommended serving size is a palm-size portion.

SMART CARBS
Carbohydrates are vital for energy production since all your cells are fueled by them. The recommended serving size is a fist-size portion.

SMART FATS
Smart fats help keep you feeling full longer and maintain healthy cholesterol levels already in the normal range. The recommended serving size is a thumb-size portion.

SMART VEGETABLES
Vegetables fortify your body with vitamins, minerals and fiber. The recommended serving size is two fist-size portions.

of food you're talking about. I'll give it to you super-quick: For protein, a portion is the size of your palm. A portion of carbs is the size of your fist. Two fists make up the size of a veggie portion. And a portion of fats is the size of your thumb. All told, on low-carb days you should be eating a total of around 1,200 calories if you're a woman and 1,500 calories if you're a man; the numbers go up to 1,500 and 2,000, respectively, on high-carb days. That's all I'll say right now, because this chapter's about cycling strategies, not food. For more on portion size and calorie counts of different foods, go to Chapter 6, "Feed Your Fire: The Recipes."

Let me simplify all this info in a chart (opposite) that sums up the fundamentals of high- and low-carb days, short and sweet.

You can see in this chart that I talk about "smart" foods. We've selected carb-cycling foods that are, well, smarter to eat than others. (Chapter 3, "Weight Loss 101," and Chapter 6, "Feed Your Fire," have everything you need to know about smart foods.) It might seem like a lot to digest, but it really isn't if you use my schedules and food lists to guide you through your low- and high-carb days. If you want to keep it as simple as possible, you can just follow these and trust that I've got the backstory right. Sure, it helps to know *why and how* carb cycling works, but the real key is to *do it*. So I won't get into all that again here; I want to get right into how you put low- and high-carb days together to create *cycling strategies*.

Cycling Specifications

Carb cycling doesn't ask anything of you that you can't handle, but do you need to follow a few rules. Any day you're carb cycling:

- Eat five meals.
- Eat within thirty minutes of waking and every three hours thereafter.
- Include both protein and carbs in your breakfast.
- Choose the right food combinations and portion sizes for *you*, given in Chapter 6, "Feed Your Fire: The Recipes."
- Drink a gallon of water daily.

Start the Day Off Right

Just like your mom told you, breakfast really is the most important meal of the day—but probably not for the reasons she thought. No matter if it's a low-carb day or a high-carb day, breakfast will *jump-start* your metabolism first thing in the morning and prime your body for a whole day of weight loss. So what if you can't eat within thirty minutes of waking up? For instance, what if you have to take medication first thing in the morning and can't have food for half an hour or an hour afterward? No problem! Just eat breakfast as soon as you possibly can. Once you do, your metabolic clock starts ticking and you keep the normal three-hour intervals between your next four meals.

Here's the Fun Part!

Before we go any farther, I want to bring you back to an incredibly important part of my carb-cycling program: rewards. These are a break in your carb-cycling routine, when I ask you to *enjoy anything you want, in moderation.* Anything! I give you two ways to claim your rewards depending on your cycle. You either get a *reward day* once a week, when you can indulge some of your food cravings throughout the day, or you get one *reward meal* on each of your high-carb days. Pretty generous, right?

Why should you stray from the straight and narrow with a reward meal or a reward day? Because believe it or not, it *keeps you on* the straight and narrow! If you can relax with your favorite foods once in a while, it's easier to follow the rules on your low- and high-carb days. Like I always say, if you can't have it now, you can have it later.

Rewards aren't exactly about the fat-melting objectives of carb cycling, but they play a powerful supporting role. Reward days and reward meals are designed to satisfy your *psychological and emotional* cravings for the sugary or fatty foods you love the most. Nothing is off limits. Nothing at all, because I don't want you to feel deprived or restricted! If you did, chances are you'd eventually fall off the carb-cycling rails—say, on an especially rough day at work or home—and then punish yourself for it or give up carb cycling altogether. When this happens, the mental consequences are a lot more damaging to your progress than the physical effects.

Another thing: I have an ulterior motive in giving you reward days. They actually help skyrocket your metabolism! Your body will raise its metabolic rate in response to the increase in calories on reward days, and hang on to that boost for some time. When you drop back into carb cycling, your calorie deficit—the difference between the number of calories you eat and the number of calories you use—is even bigger, giving you greater fat loss! *Eat what you want and still lose weight*: It's a win-win situation.

From this point forward, think of reward days and reward meals as a bonus for *a job well done*, and a necessity for your long-term success. When you pick up that burger or sit down to that slice of pie, you can give yourself a high five and say, "I've been eating clean. I've really been doing my low- and high-carb days, and I'm losing weight. I'm keeping my promises to myself! And you know what? I'm going to give myself a pat on the back and the reward I truly deserve."

Collecting Your Rewards

When you get your rewards depends on which carb-cycling plan you choose to follow. Later in this chapter I lay out four distinct cycling options, which I've designed to meet the *various needs* of different kinds of carb cyclers. That includes your need for the rich foods you love.

First, let's talk about reward *days*. I've designed three of my cycles—Classic, Turbo, and Fit—to take you into carb cycling quickly, so you can start losing weight pronto. These cycles include that once-a-week reward day, *a goal to shoot for* during your week's six low- and high-carb days. Reward days, naturally, are high-carb days, due to the kinds of foods you'll be consuming. I've made Sunday the reward day in the programs that follow, but if there is another day of the week that would be a better reward day for your life, you can declare it your reward day. But be sure you set this reward day in stone so you don't find yourself "chasing the reward"—or justifying more than one reward day a week.

Now, let's talk about reward *meals*. If you're a little hesitant and want to ease into the program slowly, I recommend you follow the Easy Cycle, which allows you to eat a reward meal on each of your four weekly high-carb days. This helps you get through the week with *frequent rewards* so you

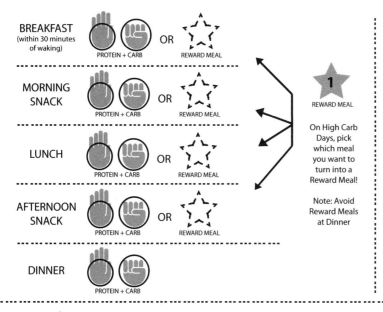

EASY CARB CYCLE - REWARD MEALS
On High Carb days, pick when you'd like to enjoy your Reward Meal

BREAKFAST (within 30 minutes of waking)
PROTEIN + CARB **OR** REWARD MEAL

MORNING SNACK
PROTEIN + CARB **OR** REWARD MEAL

LUNCH
PROTEIN + CARB **OR** REWARD MEAL

AFTERNOON SNACK
PROTEIN + CARB **OR** REWARD MEAL

DINNER
PROTEIN + CARB

1 REWARD MEAL

On High Carb Days, pick which meal you want to turn into a Reward Meal!

Note: Avoid Reward Meals at Dinner

MEALS (Eat every 3 hours and include 2 handfuls of veggies with each meal)

VEGETABLES

REWARD MEAL

Enjoy your favorite foods during your reward meal. Try not to go overboard, but ensure that you've satisfied your cravings. The more "control" you have during the Reward Meal, the quicker you'll experience weight loss. Consider enjoying your favorite foods outside of your home to keep the temptations out of your kitchen.

SMART PROTEINS

Protein is essential for weight loss since it helps build muscle. The recommended serving size is a palm-size portion.

SMART CARBS

Carbohydrates are vital for energy production since all your cells are fueled by them. The recommended serving size is a fist-size portion.

SMART FATS

Smart fats help keep you feeling full longer and maintain healthy cholesterol levels already in the normal range. The recommended serving size is a thumb-size portion.

SMART VEGETABLES

Vegetables fortify your body with vitamins, minerals and fiber. The recommended serving size is two fist-size portions.

can satisfy your cravings without cheating. With this approach, you never feel deprived. You won't mess up, so it'll be easier to keep carb cycling.

You'll learn more about all this in the rundowns of the four carb cycles, but for now I'll give you a handy chart (see opposite page) that recaps the reward basics.

Proceed With Caution

Before you go food-crazy, though, I want you to do some soul searching. Ask yourself if anything you crave might be a slippery-slope food for you that you can't stop eating once you get that first taste. Those are your *trigger foods*, and they can send your appetite and commitment into a tailspin! You should probably avoid those foods, to keep your rewards from turning into setbacks.

If you can't shake a hankering for your trigger foods, explore other options that might satisfy your needs. Say you can't resist potato chips. Try a different crunchy, salty snack, like pretzels or popcorn, instead. Pulling a switcheroo like this lets you *satisfy your appetite* while staying in control! Not every substitute will be a grand slam for your taste buds, but at least keep trying various options. If you need some ideas, check out our list of reward foods in Appendix C. Chances are, you'll find something you enjoy *even more* than your old comfort food! You'll most likely eat a little better, and you'll stay off the slippery slope to trouble. Swapping out risky foods for safer—but still tasty—ones is a wonderful tactic for taking back your power over food instead of giving it power over you. Heck, carb cycling is all about tricking your body, so why not pull one more fast one?

Carb Cycling Works for *Everyone*

Now that you know what goes into a carb-cycling day, let's find out how to turn those days into carb-cycling weeks. Depending on what you're looking to accomplish and how fast you want to do it, there are all kinds

Carb Confusion

"Chris," you might be saying, "How can I eat a bunch of carbs and lose weight?" I understand why you're worried. Everywhere you look, you get the message that carbs are bad for you and that you should cut them out altogether. The fact of the matter, though, is that carbs are *amazing* for your body! Carbohydrates are your body's super-premium fuel, and without that fuel your body won't run properly.

That's the key: *super-premium* fuel. You've got to eat the right kinds of carbs to keep your body purring. More often than not, we find ourselves eating the wrong carbs, and too much of them! Processed and refined carbohydrates—the bad stuff, like table sugar and refined flour—break down rapidly in your body, spiking your blood sugar and then crashing it. This causes uncontrollable cravings, which leads to overeating and a downward spiral. Can you guess what happens when your body takes in too many carbs? Your body ends up storing all those extra calories from carbs as *fat*.

But wait—your body's designed to run on carbohydrates! What are you supposed to do? It's a no-brainer: Eat *real*, *clean*, *natural* carbohydrates, and eat the right amount. Whole grains, beans, root vegetables, and fruits are the perfect fuel for your body. They're packed with essential vitamins and minerals. They're high in fiber, which keeps you feeling full and satisfied for a long time, without triggering cravings. You digest them more slowly, so they raise your metabolism and keep it going. Good carbs are *superfoods*. They taste great, they make you feel great, and they're great fuel for your fat-burning metabolism!

of ways to split up your week into high-carb and low-carb days (with reward days sprinkled in!). But you don't have to figure out what'll work best for you, because I've done all the heavy lifting for you! I've designed *four incredibly effective cycles*, and you get to choose the one that meets your needs. These cycles let you do all kinds of amazing things with your body, to upgrade it however you want—especially by losing weight. Awesome!

Shift Shock

Timing your meals can be confusing if you work odd hours. Carb cycling for shift workers is easy: No matter what time you wake up, aim to eat within thirty minutes, and then eat every three hours thereafter until you either go to bed or reach five meals for the day. Even if you sleep different hours on different days, keep the pattern: Eat within thirty minutes of waking and every three hours after. It couldn't be less complicated.

No matter who you are, I've got a seven-day carb cycle that fits your lifestyle and your goals. Each one of us has a unique personality, a demanding schedule, family and work circumstances that might be less than perfect, and, of course, our own individual desires and dreams. Carb cycling may not work for you unless you can *customize* it to fit into your everyday life. Maybe you just have to have a little chocolate now and then but still want to lose weight. Maybe you're in a competitive basketball league and need to maintain peak performance. Maybe you're so sick and tired of the way you look and feel that you want to kick butt and lose your butt as fast as you can.

What would you say if I told you carb cycling can do all of these things? I'm handing you the tools, and you can do *anything* you want with them!

Four Cycles, Four Goals

In my first book, *Choose to Lose*, I introduced you to my original carb cycle and outlined some variations so you could adapt carb cycling to your needs. That one-week cycle works so well that I'm bringing it back in this book, so even if you didn't read *Choose to Lose*, you can learn what it's all about. But the basic cycle might not line up with your situation, or maybe you've already been using it and you're ready to move on. That's why I've developed three more carb cycles that focus on three *specific goals*—the ones that my clients most often ask me about. Whatever you're hoping to achieve with carb cycling, one—or more!—of my four carb cycles will work for you.

You might be like a lot of other people and feel most comfortable going into a weight-loss program slow and easy. If that's where you're at, the *Easy Cycle* gives you more room to *eat your favorite foods* before you take any scary steps away from them—*if* you decide to take those steps at all. On every high-carb day you get a reward meal to eat whatever you want! And you get four high-carb days a week. Yum. You can stick with the Easy Cycle all the way down to your target weight, or you can switch to a faster cycle once you get used to the program and closer to your goal.

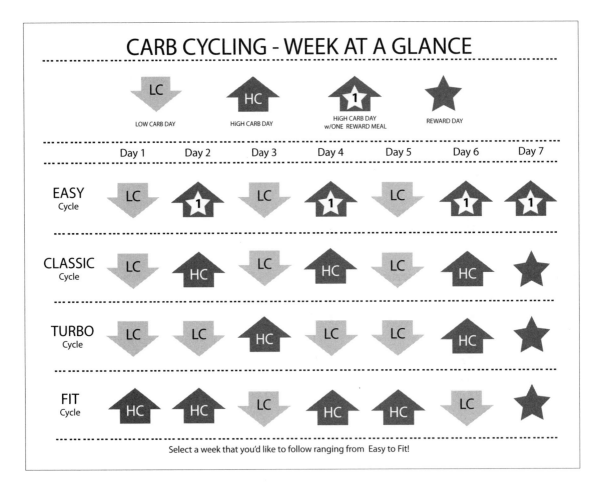

The *Classic Cycle* is where my program began, as I laid it out in *Choose to Lose*. Here, you get the straight seven-day plan that goes low-high-low-high-low-high-reward. Following this cycle is a wonderful way to learn about carb cycling, discover what it feels like, and determine how to fit it into your everyday life. Most people find that it's a good place to begin, and they like the *quick results*. It's dependable carb cycling that'll strip those inches off like nobody's business!

If you just can't stand it anymore and want to drop your excess pounds ASAP, step up to the *Turbo Cycle*, an *extreme fat-burner* that gives you two low-carb days for every high-carb day, plus one reward day a week. It's not for everyone, but boy, does it trim you down on the double! A lot of people feel fantastic on this cycle, which gives them the chance to demand the most of themselves and grab victory after victory. Not to mention that rapid weight loss. What a high!

You already challenge yourself every day if you're a serious athlete, so you've got what it takes to do a little more. If you're looking to *lean up* and drop a few pounds while still maintaining—or even enhancing—your optimal performance, you've come to the right place. The *Fit Cycle* regime flips the Turbo Cycle on its head, giving you two high-carb days for every low-carb day, plus that delicious reward day. It keeps your energy up so you can perform, and still get *ripped*!

What's My Carb Cycle?

Maybe after reading this quick rundown of the four carb cycles you know which cycle you're going to follow. But maybe you're kind of confused. Maybe you're even thinking, "Hey! I want all the benefits of all the cycles!" But you know you can only do one cycle at a time, so you're wondering, "Which cycle should I pick?" Let me help you narrow it down: Fill out the short questionnaire below to figure out which carb cycle will work the best for you.

THE RIGHT CARB CYCLE FOR ME				
If this statement is true . . . ↓	. . . circle the X's in its row ↓			
I've been able to stick with a diet in the past.		X	X	
I want a more structured plan.		X	X	
I want rapid weight loss.			X	
I want to lose weight but reward myself regularly.	X			
I choose to lose, but slow and steady is my pace.	X			X
I am very active and need sufficient energy.				X
I am training for an athletic event, but I want to lose weight.				X
I'm not very active at all.	X			
I tend to yo-yo diet and I want to stop.	X	X	X	X
I've gotten pretty good results with diets I've tried before.		X	X	
The original *Choose to Lose* cycle worked for me.		X		
I've already hit my target, and I want to maintain my new weight.	X			X
I just want to feel healthier, but I don't need to lose weight.				X
How many X's did I circle in each column (add 'em up)?				
The biggest number shows the right carb cycle for me!	Easy	Classic	Turbo	Fit

The Seven-Day Easy Cycle with Frequent Rewards

Millions of people have tried and failed and tried and failed to lose weight, and have yet to make it. Why? Because it was *just impossible* for them to give up their favorite foods for more than a week or two. Maybe you're one of those people, and you can't stand the thought of denying yourself all of the yummy stuff out there. For this very reason you're convinced you'll never be able to stick with a diet. You're afraid to even try, because it'll wreck you to try and fail yet again.

But guess what? Carb cycling, especially the Easy Cycle, lets you achieve incredible weight-loss results without saying good-bye to the foods you love! We're talking bacon. *We're talking brownies and cheesecake and gelato.* That's what the Easy Cycle is all about, so there's no reason to be scared. You *will* be able to get going and keep going with it—without feeling deprived or hemmed in.

With the Easy Cycle, if you can't have it today, you can always have it tomorrow. You get to *indulge every other day*, on your high-carb days. I have yet to meet anyone who tells me, "Gosh, I can't do this, you know, I can't wait till tomorrow." I know you *can.*

All of a sudden, dieting tastes good. Even better, you'll still lose weight! Will you lose it as quickly as you would on the other three carb cycles? Probably not. But you can feel confident that you'll finally be able to slim down without feeling deprived.

How is this even possible? Well, when it comes to junk foods, you'll be eating what you always have, but you're going to eat less of it. For example, if you're used to eating seven servings of ice cream a week, you can still eat four servings (one on each of your high-carb days, of course). On the low-carb days, you'll keep your healthier nutrition dialed in, and that fat is just going to melt right off. So you better believe you're going to see incredible results right away!

The Easy Cycle week is a simple alternating pattern of low- and high-carb days, with an extra high-carb day thrown in. The low-carb days are just like the low-carb days in the other three carb cycles, but the high-carb days . . . they're a lot more fun!

On those four wonderful high-carb days each week, you get to pick one meal—except dinner—as your reward meal. We avoid rewards at dinner because late nights tend to be a slippery slope for most. Once we start rewarding, we can't stop!

Start your lunch with a salad and blue cheese dressing, follow with a sausage-and-peppers sub, and finish your meal off with a chocolate chip cookie. I don't care! But challenge yourself to order the small or half servings instead of the medium or large, and try one cookie instead of two. You're already going to be eating additional calories on these days, so see if you can limit them. The more you do, the faster you reach your goal.

This is what your week looks like:

EASY CYCLE CARB SCHEDULE						
Monday	Tuesday	Wednesday	Thursday	Friday	Saturday	Sunday
Low-Carb	High-Carb with Reward Meal	Low-Carb	High-Carb with Reward Meal	Low-Carb	High-Carb	High-Carb with Reward Meal

Even if you're severely craving-challenged, you *can* lose weight on the Easy Cycle. But even more importantly, you're going to *prove* to yourself that you can do it. When that starts to happen, the magic ingredient of transformation—believing in yourself—reemerges and you realize, "I can do this!" That's the power of the Easy Cycle: It makes it possible for *everyone* to lose weight, to succeed with a diet, and to relearn how to believe in him- or herself.

I can't think of a bigger benefit to get from a weight-loss program, especially if you need to learn how to *believe in yourself again*. That faith and self-confidence will empower you to do anything you set out to do—not

Chasing the Diet

"Oh, no! I cheated on my low-carb day!" Don't freak out—it happens to everyone. And everyone wonders if they should make up for their slip by changing their next day to a low-carb day. The answer is no! *Never* play catch-up when it comes to your carb cycle. It'll just derail your weight-loss plan again—faster than before. You'll end up chasing your diet all over the place. Leave your mistakes in the past, where they belong. Now Confess, Reassess, and Recommit (see Chapter 2, "The True Secret of Transformation"). Face forward and keep going with your cycle . . . because you're worth it.

just lose weight! You can take that confidence and transition to a faster carb cycle, or just stick with the Easy Cycle through your whole journey to your goal. And you *will* reach your goal. It might take a little time, but hey, this is the rest of your life!

The Seven-Day Classic Cycle for Quick Results

This is where it all began, back in my first book, *Choose to Lose*. So it makes sense that the Classic Cycle is the *simplest* carb cycle of all, even though the Easy Cycle is *easier*. I designed the Classic Cycle to give you a fast and easy introduction to carb cycling. A lot of carb cyclers start their weight-loss journey with the Classic Cycle, and they stick with it because they're losing weight quickly and steadily. I've seen this cycle work for so many people, and for them, as the saying goes, "if it ain't broke, don't fix it."

The Classic Cycle is a great program if you want fast results on the scale using clear and simple guidelines. All you've got to do on the Classic Cycle is alternate low- and high-carb days six days a week, and give yourself a reward day on the seventh. Nothing complicated about it.

You're going to lose some serious weight on the Classic Cycle, and pretty quickly. But one of the great things about this cycle is that it allows you to really feel the difference in what happens to your body when you take in carbs on your high-carb days versus fats on your low-carb days. Those feelings are your body telling you what's happening as it's going through the process of weight loss. Listen to your body while you carb cycle, and you'll develop terrific body awareness. You'll actually feel the effects your food has on your body, from your energy level to your mental

CLASSIC CYCLE CARB SCHEDULE						
Monday	Tuesday	Wednesday	Thursday	Friday	Saturday	Sunday
Low-Carb	High-Carb	Low-Carb	High-Carb	Low-Carb	High-Carb	Reward

Mixed Feelings

Because you've been eating junk food, particularly high-sugar high-fat foods, for years your body is very likely to have a physical dependency on some of them. It's common to feel a bit uneasy when you first start to carb cycle and reduce your intake of these foods. Your body may go through a period of *detoxification*, when you might experience nausea, headaches, low energy, and other yucky symptoms as you remove junk foods from your diet. Don't worry, this too shall pass! However, if your detox symptoms are too uncomfortable, you may want to begin with the Easy Cycle and transition later to the Classic Cycle when your detox is done and you're ready for faster results.

clarity. The Classic Cycle will give you a whole new appreciation for the fuel you put into your body!

The Seven-Day Turbo Cycle for Rapid Weight Loss

Are you ready to shed your extra padding *fast*—as fast as you possibly can? Yes? Then this cycle is for you. The Turbo Cycle gets results the quickest—and takes off the most pounds per week—of the four carb cycles.

This cycle works like lightning because it's lean and mean. Instead of the basic one day on/one day off carb cycle, the Turbo Cycle puts two low-carb days up against every high-carb day. You've got two fat-burning days for every metabolism-stoking day, so you slim down really, really fast.

While the Turbo Cycle gives you the fastest results of any carb cycle, it's *not* a severely restricted-calorie diet that'll crash your metabolism. Women: Don't consume fewer than 1,200 calories a day! Men: Don't consume fewer than 1,500 calories! You'll still get results very quickly. The Turbo Cycle is totally safe and incredibly effective!

TURBO CYCLE CARB SCHEDULE						
Monday	Tuesday	Wednesday	Thursday	Friday	Saturday	Sunday
Low-Carb	Low-Carb	High-Carb	Low-Carb	Low-Carb	High-Carb	Reward

On the Turbo Cycle, you're going to get results in no time, but there's a trade-off you should know about. With two low-carb days in a row, you're definitely going to feel a dip in your energy level—especially on that second day—but it's a clear sign that you're losing inches. And just watch how rapidly the numbers on your scale go down. Those low-carb days are powerful weight-loss accelerators.

The Seven-Day Fit Cycle for Athletic Performance

If you have an active lifestyle and you want to lean up *without compromising* your athletic performance, the Fit Cycle is a great option. Like a lot of other diets, the Fit Cycle strips off your fat, but unlike most of them it also supplies the fuel you need to excel in your sport of choice or to train for long stretches of time each day.

Of all the four cycles I lay out in this chapter, the Fit Cycle includes the fewest low-carb days: only two per week. I've got you *eating more carbs* so you can drive more of them into your muscles, filling them up with fuel. As an athlete, you probably know that those carbs get converted to glucose, then are stored in your muscle as glycogen. That's the stuff your muscles tap when they need energy, so if you want maximum physical performance you will need those glycogen stores. Score one for the Fit Cycle!

What you might not know is that a really cool thing happens when athletes carb cycle. On your low-carb days, when you deplete your glycogen stores, your muscles develop *insulin sensitivity*. So what, you say? Well, when you switch back over to a high-carb day, or when you enjoy your weekly reward day, your insulin-sensitive muscles do something brilliant. It's called *super-compensation*, and it means that your muscles actually soak up *more* carbs than they normally would. Your body burns the extra fuel to keep your performance high, instead of storing it as fat. Your metabolism is pumped, so taking in the extra carbs actually helps you lose weight!

Because you're in a high-carb mode, you won't be losing weight as fast as you would on the Turbo Cycle. It's the sacrifice you make to maintain your performance! In fact, structurally the Fit Cycle is the opposite of the Turbo Cycle.

FIT CYCLE CARB SCHEDULE						
Monday	Tuesday	Wednesday	Thursday	Friday	Saturday	Sunday
High-Carb	High-Carb	Low-Carb	High-Carb	High-Carb	Low-Carb	Reward

Even though it's a high-carb program, the Fit Cycle will put you at a calorie deficit for some weight loss, so you might take *a slight hit to your performance*. If you're focused on your performance and don't want to lose weight, pre- and post-workout supplementation, perhaps meal-replacement shakes with some extra macronutrients, can help fuel your performance while minimizing weight loss.

Carb Cycling Away from Home

None of us eat every meal at home. And when we're not home, we can't always take our food with us. I spend *tons* of time on the road and eat in restaurants all the time, so I've figured out a few ways to keep on carb cycling wherever I am.

My Top Four Traveling Tactics
1. Pack nonperishable items to bring with you. Whey protein powder, fruit, and nuts are good choices.

2. When you get to your destination, take a bus, taxi, or car to a grocery store on the way to your hotel and stock up on smart proteins, carbs, fats, and veggies. Most bus and taxi drivers know where to buy food along their route.
3. At your hotel, request a microwave and/or refrigerator for your room, so you can store perishable items and heat up some healthy meals.
4. Always carry a shaker bottle so you can make protein shakes.

My Top Five Restaurant Tactics
1. Drink a tall glass of water as soon as it's brought to the table. If your server doesn't pour water automatically, request some. Keep drinking water throughout your meal.
2. Order your entrée grilled, broiled, baked, boiled, or steamed—never sautéed or fried.
3. Many restaurants allow you to order a side of grilled chicken, fish, or beef. Do so if you can, and select carbs and veggies from the rest of the sides menu.
4. If your dish includes sauce or dressing, ask for it on the side.
5. Split your dish with your dining partner or request half of it to go when you order. I've never had any restaurant refuse this request!

Resetting for Continued Weight Loss

Carb cycling is one of the most effective ways to keep your body guessing about what you're going to throw at it next. And as we've talked about, *faking out your body* is a powerful tool for weight loss. But no matter which carb cycle you're on, your smart body will eventually *figure out the pattern* and adapt.

Depending on your body, some reach a weight-loss plateau or slow down anytime between the fourth and twelfth weeks of carb cycling.

Most people respond to a plateau by thinking, "I just need to eat less and exercise more." Don't do it! You'll just get more firmly stuck on your plateau. And don't give up on carb cycling! Now's the time to turn the tables again, and trick your body back into losing more weight. Now's the time to use my *Slingshot Technique*.

A Slingshot is seven high-carb days in a row. Yup, I'm asking you to *eat more*. And yes, the seventh day is still a reward day! Every carb cycler should Slingshot: In fact, I consider it an essential part of carb cycling. And it's so easy! All you need to do is to *follow your carb cycle for three weeks, then take one Slingshot week*.

By adding Slingshots to your carb cycle, you're constantly changing the way you eat—a technique that we fitness professionals call *periodization*. It's incredibly effective because taking a week off from your normal carb-cycling routine fools your body all over again. Eliminate low-carb days and fuel up for a week, and you'll con your metabolism into reigniting and burning down your weight-loss wall!

High-carb days during Slingshot weeks are exactly the same as high-carb days during the cycles. Breakfast, which you eat within half an hour of getting up, is a portion of protein, a portion of carbs, and, if you want, any amount of vegetables. After that you eat four more meals, one every three hours, consisting of a portion of protein, a portion of carbs, and a portion of veggies. Eat this way for seven straight days, and enjoy yourself.

During the Slingshot, you do the same amount of exercise as you do while carb cycling. With all those high-carb days filling your muscles with fuel, you should notice that your performance increases significantly.

For as long as you're carb cycling, Slingshot for one week after every three weeks of high-carb/low-carb cycling. This technique keeps most people from plateauing at all, but if your body does adapt to the three weeks on, one week off pattern, do a Slingshot then and there to rocket off your plateau. When you do return to your normal carb cycle, you'll keep dropping pounds. You might even start losing weight faster! So don't fudge the rules. Stay on course!

And remember that everybody responds to the cycle/Slingshot model a bit differently. Your weight might stay the same for those seven days, or it might drop significantly. If you gain any weight, it's typically because you're retaining water that'll flush out of your system when you return to carb cycling. If your weight loss has been stalling, the Slingshot is usually just what your body needs to get those pounds dropping off again. However, there's a small possibility that the Slingshot will not break your plateau. If that happens, you'll need to make some other changes in your program to get the results you want:

- Check your portion sizes and fine-tune them if you need to (use the 100-calorie info in Chapter 6, "Feed Your Fire: The Recipes" as a reference).
- Try switching to a faster carb cycle: Easy to Classic, Classic to Turbo.

Weigh-ins

Weigh-ins are a great way to monitor the progress you're making. Weigh in just *once* per week, in the morning, after a low-carb day. This is when you will get the most accurate weight for your body. See next page for what a sample schedule might look like:

CARB CYCLING - BEST WEIGH IN DAYS

Weigh yourself on the MORNING of the circled day of each cycle for the most true weigh in.

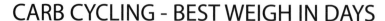

	Day 1	Day 2	Day 3	Day 4	Day 5	Day 6	Day 7
EASY Cycle	LC	1	LC	1	LC	(1)	1
CLASSIC Cycle	LC	HC	LC	HC	LC	(HC)	★
TURBO Cycle	LC	LC	HC	LC	LC	(HC)	★
FIT Cycle	HC	HC	LC	HC	HC	LC	(★)

If you feel you must weigh in multiple times a week, you will weigh less on the morning of a High Carb day that FOLLOWS a Low Carb day.

Let me explain. Your body loses fat in slow motion. When we break it all down, you may be losing one-quarter to upward of a half a pound of fat daily. This might not seem like much, but it adds up to nearly two to four pounds per week! However, the scale might not always read this way daily. While we may lose a fraction of a pound in fat each day, our bodies can also fluctuate between two and ten pounds of water! Mentally, this can be extremely frustrating when we are fixated on the number on the scale to keep us motivated.

Now let's get real. Many of you are going to weigh yourself daily, regardless of my warnings. If you do, let me explain what to expect so you don't freak out. Carbs are like magnets for water in the body, so when you eat them you will naturally find during your weigh-in that you've retained more water. Your scale should read higher the morning after high-carb days and lower the morning after low-carb days. As you go through the week following the Classic Cycle, for example, your weight may look something like this:

Monday morning—gain 3 pounds
Tuesday morning —lose 4 pounds
Wednesday morning—gain 2 pounds
Thursday morning—lose 2 pounds
Friday morning—gain 3 pounds
Saturday morning—lose 4 pounds
Sunday morning – no change.

Your weight has seesawed through the week, but overall you have lost two pounds. That's how it works!

Now, there is one popular ingredient in our foods that can throw off a weigh-in in the worst way—sodium. Sodium is like a super-magnet for water in our bodies and can hold pounds on our bodies during the weigh-in. Keep in mind that a gallon of water weighs eight pounds, and it is not uncommon for sodium to be able to hold that much in us! So if you are putting in the work and eating right, but have a weigh-in that baffles you, think back a day or two and notice how much sodium you may have eaten in canned foods, cured meats, or other processed foods. Not to worry though, just wait until next week and you should see the scale drop nicely!

As you can see, carb cycling can be as unique as you are! Choosing the cycle that is right for you isn't tough; it's fast, easy, and fun. The best part? You're in complete control and can switch to another cycle at any time, if needed. And remember, whether you're a busy mom, competitive athlete, couch potato, or businessman, *there is a cycle for you!*

5

SHAPE YOUR BODY, SHRED YOUR FAT: THE EXERCISES

A t her heaviest, Annette weighed 217 pounds. She hadn't always been overweight: In fact, once upon a time she'd been in great shape. Then she had four kids, dropped into depression, and developed allergies and breathing problems. Month after month, year after year, Annette's weight crept up and up and her health sank down and down. Too heavy and too sick, she felt lousy every minute of every day.

Bottom line, Annette didn't like herself, and she hated the way she looked. For years, she avoided the camera and wouldn't pose for pictures with her children or grandchildren. When her daughter-in-law posted pictures of a family birthday party on Facebook, Annette wanted to crawl into a hole. She tried all sorts of weight-loss strategies, from starving herself to bodybuilding, but nothing worked. If she did manage to drop some weight, she always gained it back.

Annette knew that her weight was affecting her kids. Her daughter told her that she wished she could reach all the way around her mom when they hugged. Her son carved the number of a weight-loss hotline into her nightstand. Those were flashing red lights. Struggling with exhaustion, despair, and disgust, Annette finally had her moment of clarity. She decided that she would never let her kids down again. She knew she needed to

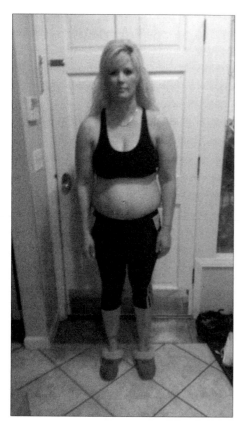

change her lifestyle—not just her body. She wanted to really *live* her life. She made a commitment to transformation.

That's when Annette found out about carb cycling and sighed to herself, "Why not?" When she started following my nutrition and exercise program, she began to feel better in only a week or two. That was strong motivation to stick with carb cycling, and she did. She ate healthy meals and began to exercise every day. She set a target weight of 135 pounds, which meant she was shooting to lose 82 pounds. Once she started carb cycling, Annette dropped 24 pounds in eleven weeks. By week fourteen she had ditched a total of 34 pounds. Now Annette maintains her weight at 134 pounds.

Exercise was the key to Annette's success. She faithfully cycled her carbs, but she really poured her heart into her workouts. At first, she focused on becoming more mobile and active in little ways—walking everywhere she could, taking the stairs instead of the elevator. When she first went back to the gym, she was upset to discover just how out of shape she was. It took incredible commitment, work, and sweat for Annette to build up her strength and endurance almost from square one.

Annette didn't give up this time. She taped a "before" picture of herself to her bathroom door to remind herself every day why she was pursuing transformation. Riding bikes and taking hikes with her kids was another reminder. In fact, Annette made fitness a family affair—and her family became her rock, encouraging her in tough times and cheering her successes.

Carb cycling has truly transformed Annette. In every way, she's a healthier, happier person. She loves herself again, she feels alive all the time, and her energy is always in high gear. Annette knows exactly how she got her life back, so she's embraced the carb-cycling lifestyle . . . for life. She still loves doing her 9-Minute Missions first thing five mornings a week; they're such a great start to her day. She still loves her Shredders six days a week; they give her amazing get-up-and-go. What's next? Annette wants to lose five more pounds, tone up to the max, and enter a figure competition! Rock on, Annette!

Annette's determination is humbling. She isn't much different from the next person, but no matter what weight-loss or fitness plateaus she hits, she keeps powering through to her transformation goals. She wants it so much that even when she feels like she can't push her workout any farther, she'll do one more rep or walk one more mile—and maybe another, and another—and it makes her feel fantastic.

A lot of my other clients have discovered the same thing. For them, carb cycling is about so much more than losing weight. And, like Annette, many of my clients choose to concentrate on the exercise component of the carb-cycling program. You'll be amazed to see how effective these exercises are, and to see where your mind and body can take you if you go with their flow. Trust the program. It works!

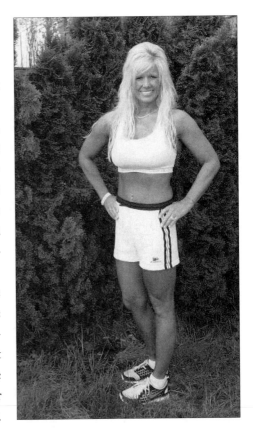

Build Up and Break Through!

Your body is made to move! It's made to push, pull, squat, crunch, run, jump, and climb. And that's just what I'm going to show you how to do, so you can blaze through fat at an insane rate *and* get fit.

Your body is the most faithful companion you'll ever have. Wherever you go, no matter what you do, it'll be there with you. Its love is unconditional, but you've still got to treat it right if you want it to stick around. You're *the only one* who can do that: It's 100 percent dependent on you for all its needs. Think of your body almost like a pet—you've got to feed it good, natural food (not too much!); make sure it's got plenty of fresh water; and let it play and run and jump. Your body *wants* to move and be healthy, and when you take good care of it, it'll help you achieve your goals: to lose weight, increase your energy and mental clarity, and enrich your quality of life. Get moving, and you'll feel pretty darn great!

It's astounding what exercise can do for you. Sure, it makes you stronger and beautifully sculpts your body, but there's a whole lot more to it. Exercise delivers nutrients to all of your cells and oxygenates your organs, tissues, and muscles, giving you *tons of energy*. More and more research shows that exercise has a powerful role in cleaning toxins out of your cells, including your brain cells. When your brain wrings out toxins and soaks up nutrients and oxygen, your mental clarity pops, your depression evaporates, and your productivity skyrockets! Oh, and did I mention that exercise burns right through those extra pounds?

There are so many fantastic upsides to exercise. You want to know how many downsides there are? Zero. It's guaranteed: The more you move, the better your life. Exercise *transforms* your life!

The Fast Track to a Lean *and* Fit Body

Carb cycling lays the foundation for weight loss, but exercise accelerates the process, producing outstanding results on the double. Combine nutrition and exercise, and you throw a one-two punch at your fat. That's why exercise is an essential factor if you want to drop a lot of pounds in a little time. But I not only want you to lose weight, *I want you to be fit!* I want you to have a beautifully functioning body that lasts your whole life. So I'm going to show you the two steps to getting fit while losing weight.

But first, I have to tell you something fantastic: To get fit, you don't have to join a health club. You don't need to buy expensive equipment. And you definitely don't need to order the contraptions you see in TV advertisements and stores. In fact, you don't need much more than your own body: It's your *incredible, built-in, private gym*. Your body, a floor, and a chair are all you need to do your 9-Minute Missions; depending on what kind of Shredders you choose, you might also need to pick up a few basics like a pair of sneakers or a bathing suit.

Not only is your gym inexpensive and simple to use—it's portable. You take your body *wherever you go*, so you can work out whether you're at home or on the road. Talk about user-friendly! I'm going to show you how to use your fully equipped, conveniently located gym to get the results you're after. You're about to discover how easy it is to make exercise an enjoyable lifestyle and to stay youthful, lose fat, and get fit.

START EACH WEEKDAY WITH YOUR 9-MINUTE MISSION

I can just hear you asking, "What the heck is a 9-Minute Mission?" Simply put, they are the workouts that *shape and develop your muscles*. Some people call this kind of exercise resistance training or strength training. My version centers on three of the most fundamental movements of the human body: pushing, crunching, and squatting.

I've taken a bunch of muscle-building exercises and designed a series of quick, convenient 9-Minute Missions for you to do one of when you wake up in the morning Monday through Friday. The missions are a challenge, but when you accomplish them, the results are profound. You get energy and a boosted metabolism, as well as increased fat loss, muscle development, and brain oxygenation—the list goes on!

9-Minute Missions boost your metabolism like crazy by stimulating and growing your *energy-hungry muscles*. Not only will you use a whole lot of calories while you're exercising, but your oxygen-depleted, pumped-up muscles will munch through carbs and fat *for the rest of the day*. 9-Minute Missions will always give you results, but you'll be amazed at how much better they work when you do them first thing in the morning. Five days a week, these nine minutes of fast, fun, high-intensity morning exercise speed up your weight loss. Start your day right, and you're set for a whole day of burning fat and feeling great—even if you're stuck in a cubicle at work.

If you read my first book, *Choose to Lose*, you'll remember the three powerful 9-Minute Mission workouts I gave you (I called them Shapers). I got such incredible feedback on those that I want to give you more this time. I'm going to show you just how creative we can get with running, jumping, pushing, crunching, and squatting. Now you'll have twenty entirely new, incredibly powerful 9-Minute Missions to use in your transformation. Cycle through them and watch the immense increase in your fitness!

DO A SHREDDER LATER IN THE DAY

You can accelerate your fat loss even more by adding *Shredders* to your exercise program. I call these workouts Shredders because they turn you into a shredding machine that aggressively destroys your body fat. Shredders are cardio workouts, often called aerobic exercise, like walking, biking, and swimming. They're *interval* training that alternates periods of exercise with periods of rest. I've pulled years of my research together to design Shredders that get results in the *least amount of time* with the *least amount of effort*.

Like 9-Minute Missions, Shredders accelerate and maximize your fat loss, but you do them at a lower intensity, in longer sessions, ranging from five to sixty minutes. And you can do them any time of day, because they work differently from 9-Minute Missions: They incinerate fat *while* you exercise. As you run, row, or dance the rumba, your heart pumps faster and your blood rushes through your body, loading your organs with oxygen and converting the padding on your hips and belly into energy *right then and there*. Like an ice cube in the hot sun, your fat melts away. Talk about motivation to work out!

I've made a few changes to the Shredders since I introduced them in *Choose to Lose*. I've made them easier! Easier to follow, that is. While the impact of alternating low-, medium-, and high-intensity is phenomenal, sometimes it's difficult to gauge your intensity levels. That's why this time around I've created four different Shredders with just two levels of intensity: low and high. Super-simple, super-easy to follow. No more guesswork!

Your Workouts of the Day

My exercise program sets you up with a 9-Minute Mission and a Shredder for each weekday. Combining their power, the program does two jobs:

burns fat and increases fitness. Heck, if you're putting in the time, you might as well kill two birds with one stone! You can sharpen your aim when you throw that stone by doing your Shredder and 9-Minute Mission workouts *at set times every day*: 9-Minute Missions first thing in the morning and Shredders anytime afterward, at whatever time you establish for yourself.

I know you're going to stick with the schedule you set and actually do your exercises, because I've designed the 9-Minute Missions and Shredders to be fun. I want you to look forward to your workouts! Fitness is a game you play with yourself, a challenge you'll want to meet. You'll be excited to reach weight-loss and fitness pinnacles that you've never thought you could reach, and to push the envelope of your potential.

You're going to love your 9-Minute Missions, because they're such a fun and easy way to win a victory first thing in the morning. It's so fulfilling to *give your all to yourself* before you do anything else each day. Immediately after your 9-Minute Mission, or in the afternoon or evening, you'll have a blast with your Shredders, because you'll be doing an activity that you truly love. If you *like what you're doing*, you're going to keep doing it. You don't have to jog for your cardio if you hate to jog—take a class or play some basketball instead if you like to. Enjoy yourself, and transform your life at the same time.

One Size Doesn't Fit All

Whether you've been a couch potato for years or you're a well-conditioned athlete, my exercise program will work for you. That's because it's scalable—*you can gear your workout to your fitness level*. A 9-Minute Mission or twenty minutes of Shredding can be daunting if you haven't moved a muscle in ages, so if you're just starting out, you can take it slowly. Even if you're athletic, high-intensity 9-Minute Missions and Shredders can be challenging. But if you're already active, you can find the higher level that's right for you—and go for it! Either way, you'll fire up your metabolism and maximize your weight-loss potential.

The beauty of the 9-Minute Missions is that they're based on *your* ability level. When the clock starts, you simply do what *you* are capable of doing. Your performance the first time you do a mission sets your baseline, and it only goes up from there! It's so fun when you repeat a Mission from the previous month and see how much your performance has increased. You can literally *see and feel* the proof that your fitness is going up!

If you're just starting out with exercise, follow the beginner or intermediate versions of the exercises laid out below until you master them and feel comfortable trying the more advanced movements . . . but don't rush it! Keep your speed controlled as you get a feel for the movement and timing of each Mission. As you begin to feel more and more comfortable, increase your speed. The fitter you get, the faster you go!

Wake Up and Shape Up: Your 9-Minute Missions

I love to start out my day with a 9-Minute Mission. It's convenient, and it makes the most of that *quick burst* of high-intensity strength training. 9-Minute Missions sculpt and develop your muscles and definitely improve your physique, plus—they're stamina-building machines! But their bigger benefit for weight loss is that they get you ready to incinerate fat. By putting your muscles in motion, the 9-Minute Missions totally hyperactivate your fat- and carb-burning mechanisms, so you lose weight on the double!

9-Minute Mission workouts spur your muscles to devour tons of carbs, so your body ends up with a lot fewer carbs to store as fat. Your 9-Minute Missions also *fire up your metabolism* to melt the fat that your body's already stored. Plus, 9-Minute Missions build and preserve your muscles to drive your metabolism even harder. A bonus upside is that these high-power workouts dose your bloodstream with a hormone that increases fat eradication even more. I'm not kidding!

It's awesome! 9-Minute Missions accelerate your weight loss in *four great ways*:

1. No New Fat!

When you put your muscles through short, intense workouts like the 9-Minute Missions, they empty their own energy reserves before they start drawing on your body fat. Muscles store energy in the form of glycogen, a converted form of carbohydrate. Your 9-Minute Mission workout drains glycogen from your muscles, leaving them hungry for more carbs. You've got a glycogen deficit, an energy hole you've got to fill. That's one reason to do your resistance training first thing in the morning: The carbs you eat at breakfast will *be soaked up into your muscles as glycogen.* That's right: You should eat carbs at breakfast.

What happens if you eat oatmeal or toast or hash browns when your muscles are already full of carbs (maybe because you haven't done your 9-Minute Mission . . .)? Some of it's used by your working muscles and organs, but the rest of the glucose that's broken down from the carbs doesn't have anywhere to go, so your body stores it as fat. But the solution isn't simply to stop eating carbs: Even if you're just sitting around, your muscles, and all of your organs, *need that fuel*—and they need a lot more of it when you're in motion. If you don't eat carbs, your body will panic and try to preserve its fuel supply—your fat. So, as I mentioned in Chapter 4, to burn fat, you've actually got to eat carbs!

But before you eat the carbs you have to do your 9-Minute Missions. Working your muscles fast and furious before taking in carbs will force your muscles to soak the carbs right up. There's nothing left to store as fat, so your fat can't grow. What's more, the effect of doing your 9-Minute Missions lasts *for the rest of the day.* Pretty cool! It's a tactic I've used for years to help my clients take control of their body and their weight.

2. A Fierce Metabolism

You can control your nutrition, too, to control your metabolism and create an even bigger carb deficit. When you eat carbs after doing your 9-Minute Missions, the glucose that you drive into your muscles ends up exactly where we want it. By pumping new fuel into them, boom! *those muscles roar to life.* Carbs are like ninety-two-octane—no, one-hundred-octane—gas for your internal combustion engine. Your muscles instantly go from zero to sixty, spiking your metabolism.

That metabolic combustion *keeps going for hours* after you do your 9-Minute Missions. The oxygen in your blood goes on combining with the glycogen in your muscles to ignite your metabolism again and again. Your muscles keep burning through their energy reserves, so they're starving for more carbs. Muscles are very greedy, and when it comes to nutrition your body gives them priority over other organs—and over fat. A lot more nutrient-rich blood travels through muscle than through fat, so if your muscles are fired up by 9-Minute Missions, they gobble up the carbs *before* those calories reach your fat.

3. Hot Muscles

You need an insurance policy for a high-performance machine like your muscles. The 9-Minute Missions are that insurance: By stimulating your muscles to grow, the Missions protect your muscles from cannibals. *What?!* Well, for most people who are trying to trim down, losing fat means losing some muscle in the process, too. That's right: Their bodies end up cannibalizing a lot of muscle, in addition to fat, for energy. And since muscles are the body's biggest carb burners, people who shrink their muscles slow down their metabolism. You know what *that* means!

You can't afford to lose any of your precious muscle, because it's your metabolic engine. Doing just a few minutes of vigorous resistance training really helps spare your muscles—by rebuilding them. Your body's just like everyone else's, so if you're working out almost every day, your metabolism will go after your muscles for energy. But by doing your 9-Minute Missions, you keep rebuilding your muscles, so even if you lose some, you gain more. You come out ahead! Your metabolic engine doesn't break down, and you keep burning calories like crazy. Fantastic! It's essential to keep your metabolism as high as possible so you can *maintain your weight loss for the rest of your life*. 9-Minute Missions can help you do that.

4. A Secret Weapon

Now here's your bonus: 9-Minute Missions *keep you looking young*. Wow! The brief, high-intensity running, jumping, pushing, squatting, and crunching of 9-Minute Mission exercises trigger a sensational neuroendocrine response. That's a fancy way of saying that your workouts tell your brain to release some incredible hormone called growth hormone. And let me tell you, that stuff is like liquid gold.

When you do your 9-Minute Missions, you tap into a real-world fountain of youth! In nine minutes a day you start your growth hormone flowing. That miracle juice attacks fat, which is great—the more the merrier, when it comes to anti-fat weapons. But the real gravy is that growth hormone replenishes your cells. Big deal, you say? Yeah, it is. This stuff makes you *grow new cells when your old ones die.*

Young cells keep you healthy and looking young. Have you ever noticed that a lot of hard-core fitness buffs look more youthful than other folks their age? It's not just because they're in great shape: It's because they've found their very own fountains of youth. You can, too, by doing *short bursts of intense exercise*—your 9-Minute Missions—which pump growth hormone into your veins, constantly rejuvenating your body. Believe it!

Five Ways to Do Your 9-Minute Missions

Here's where I give you the phenomenal techniques you'll be using to put the pedal to your weight-loss metal—to set your body's four powerful metabolic mechanisms in motion. I've created *twenty new 9-Minute Mission workouts built on thirty original exercises* that go beyond the ones I showed you in my first book. (I'll take you through those thirty exercises step-by-step after I lay out the twenty workouts here.) But don't worry if you didn't read *Choose to Lose*. Newbies can totally rock these exercises.

Having thirty new exercises and twenty new workouts to choose from will *keep your routine fresh* and exciting. Plus, I've shaved a minute off my original *ten-minute* rule. Nine minutes give you the exact same results as ten minutes, so I've saved you a whole extra minute of work! Who doesn't have nine minutes?

You'll be doing a totally different 9-Minute Mission—giving your body a totally new challenge—on each of five days a week, every week, for a month (you get two days off per week!). That's why I'm giving you exactly twenty workouts: Five 9-Minute Missions a week for four weeks = twenty 9-Minute Missions per month. You're not going to repeat a single 9-Minute Mission all month, so you sure won't get bored! And when you switch up the exercises that you use in your 9-Minute Missions from day to day, *plus* do them in the different ways I describe below, you're *really* giving your body the kind of variety that's the spice of weight loss. Your body never gets in a groove, never adapts to your resistance training regimen, so it *never stops moving forward*. Each day, each week, your muscles keep growing and your waistline keeps shrinking.

In month two, you'll do the whole cycle of twenty workouts over again, and when you do, you'll see some big changes. Going back through the 9-Minute Mission cycle and performing each workout one month after you last did it, you'll see a significant, quantifiable jump in your fitness level. You'll be able to do more reps and more circuits in the same amount of time. It's more workout for your minute: You get a bigger payoff from each and every 9-Minute Mission! And it happens again and again in months three and four and each month that follows. Outstanding.

This system keeps you breaking through your fitness and weight-loss plateaus so you can achieve the results you're looking for!

Each of the twenty 9-Minute Mission workouts is designed according to one of five protocols. For each, I give you a workout plan, a pinpointed goal, and a Breakthrough Training Tactic for taking your workout to the next level. And to help you get started, I lay out four great 9-Minute Missions for each of the five protocols. Each Mission targets one of the three zones of your body—upper, core, and lower—or your total body, and it doesn't matter how many reps or how many rounds you complete in it. Whether you do two rounds or twenty rounds, five reps or fifty reps, it's nine minutes and you're done. As long as you give it your best effort, you win! It's all super-easy—so are you ready to shape up?

What's He Talking About?

Whoa. I'm using a lot of fitness jargon! This little glossary should clear up any confusion you might be experiencing.

9-Minute Mission: This is the total workout. There are five different styles of missions: Sprintervals, Stepladders, Enduros, Super Circuits, and Rapid Rounds.

Circuit: A full round of exercises in a mission, from the first exercise to the last.

Interval: A period of time during which your body is either working at specific intensities or resting. Interval training alternates these periods.

Rep: An abbreviation for *repetition*, which is a single, full completion of an exercise movement, from the first step to the last.

Rest: An interval during a workout when you aren't moving, but letting your body recover before the next interval of exercise.

Round: A circuit.

Dominating Your Inner Dialogue

While we're exercising, we all carry on an *inner dialogue* in our head. The conversation might not be in actual words, but the feelings become strong when you begin to notice your muscles burning, your heart beating faster, and your rapid breathing. Your brain immediately monitors these sensations to see if you're in danger and when you should stop exercise so you don't get injured. This sets up a struggle, because your body's discomfort typically triggers your brain to say "stop!" well before you're remotely close to injury. Many call this the *mental barrier*, and it can block you from the results you're capable of achieving. It can keep you from taking good fitness up to great fitness. But you *can* break through your mental barrier!

Doing the different 9-Minute Missions, you'll experience different physical responses. Pay attention, and you'll eventually discover your own *personal* mental barrier. In each workout description, I lay out the physical sensations you can expect. I also equip you with a *breakthrough training tactic* that you can use to blast through your mental barrier, accomplish your mission, and reach the victory (and fitness!) you deserve. By smashing your mental barrier again and again, you take back your power, to take control of your inner dialogue. When you do this day after day, your fitness skyrockets, your weight drops, and you begin to appreciate how strong you really are, both mentally and physically!

There are three steps to dominating your inner dialogue and breaking through your mental barrier:

- SEEK OUT your mental barrier: Intensify your mission until you can hear your inner dialogue clearly. Listen as your body tries to talk you into stopping. "This is hard. I can really feel the load on my muscles. I should stop before it gets uncomfortable." "The burn is getting intense. I don't know if I can stand it much longer. I should stop so the burn goes away." "My breathing is getting heavy and my heart rate is going up. I should stop and catch my breath."
- PUSH AGAINST your mental barrier: Keep going with your mission until your body's arguments become urgent. If you're anxious about the burning in your muscles, you might hear, "I'm scared! My muscles are burning so brutally! I have to stop!" If your breathing is becoming panicky, your body might be screaming, "I'm scared! I can't breathe! I have to stop or I'm going to suffocate!"
- BREAK THROUGH your mental barrier with two tactics:
  - +2 method → When you reach the point in your mission where your muscles are blazing and too fatigued to do another rep, there's a way to keep chipping away at your reps until you complete your mission. Stop and rest for five seconds, then perform two more reps. Stop again and rest for five more seconds, then do two more reps. Continue until you complete your mission.
  - Power breathing→ Your body has a natural tendency to go into hyperventilation, or *panic breathing*, but there's an extremely ef-

fective way to overcome this. The key is to keep your jaw loose and breathe aggressively through *both* your nose and mouth. Each time you inhale, try to inflate your lungs an extra "inch" at the top of the breath, then exhale quickly but not forcefully. Keep breathing like this until you complete your mission. You'll be able to remain in mental and physical control!

The Sprinterval Mission

This strategy is all about work and rest. Under this protocol, your Missions challenge and develop your muscular and cardiorespiratory endurance as well as your stamina. A 20-second burst of exercise work doesn't seem like much at first, but it becomes a real challenge in the later rounds. Focus power breathing early on, and as your muscles begin to burn out, use the +2 Method to conquer the mission!

Goal: *Do as many repetitions as possible during each interval. Keep track of your total repetitions and write them down. When you do the 9-Minute Mission next month, compare your numbers and watch your progress!*

Breakthrough Training Tactic: *power breathing and +2 method*

What You'll Need: *a stopwatch, a clock with a sweeping hand, or a smartphone app with timer*

PROTOCOL

1. Do as many repetitions as you can of Exercise #1 (see below) for 20 seconds, then rest for 10 seconds. That's a 30-second interval.
2. Repeat the interval 5 more times, for a total of 3 minutes.
3. Repeat steps 1 and 2 for Exercises #2 and #3.

There you have it: 3 exercises for 3 minutes each = a 9-Minute Mission!

Four Great Sprinterval Missions

(See the 9-Minute Missions exercise instructions following the five mission protocols for information on these exercises.)

THIGH MASTER (LOWER BODY)
Exercise #1: Back Lunge
Exercise #2: Air Squats
Exercise #3: Bridge-Ups

RUN LIKE THE WIND (TOTAL BODY)
Exercise #1: High Knees
Exercise #2: Push-Ups
Exercise #3: Back Lunge

TGIF (TOTAL BODY)
Exercise #1: Dive Bombers
Exercise #2: Knees to Elbows
Exercise #3: Air Squat

SHOULDER SHAKER (UPPER BODY)
Exercise #1: Bench Dip
Exercise #2: Pike Press
Exercise #3: Squat Thrust

The Rapid Rounds Mission

This strategy's all about short, quick circuits, performed as fast as you can, as many as you can, for 2 minutes. Each of the four Missions I outline challenges and develops your cardiorespiratory endurance, stamina, and speed—a 2-minute window is perfect for this. Don't worry about burning out, you get to rest and recover for a minute between each 2-minute surge. Use power breathing to break through your mental barrier and conquer your Mission. Once you feel comfortable and proficient with the movements, go hard and fast with this one!

Goal: *Do as many circuits as possible during each 2-minute interval.*

Breakthrough Training Tactic: *power breathing*

What You'll Need: *a stopwatch, a clock with a sweeping hand, or a smartphone app with timer*

PROTOCOL

1. Perform the set number of repetitions of Exercise #1, immediately followed by the set number of repetitions of Exercise #2 and the set number of repetitions of Exercise #3 to complete a circuit. Do as many circuits as you can in 2 minutes. Go all out! Take 1 minute of rest. That's an interval of 3 minutes.
2. Repeat the interval twice more for a total of 3 circuits.

Fantastic! 3 circuits for 3 minutes each = a 9-Minute Mission!

Four Great Rapid Rounds Missions

(See the 9-Minute Missions exercise instructions following the five Mission protocols for information on these exercises.)

FIVE ALIVE (TOTAL BODY)

Exercise #1: Burpee	5 reps
Exercise #2: Twisters	5 reps
Exercise #3: Marching Soldiers	5 reps

EASY THREEZIES (CORE)

Exercise #1: Squat Thrusts	3 reps
Exercise #2: Twisters	6 reps
Exercise #3: Swing-Ups	9 reps

JACKPOT (TOTAL BODY)

Exercise #1: Twisters	7 reps
Exercise #2: Marching Soldiers	7 reps
Exercise #3: Squat Thrusts	7 reps

SEVEN ELEVEN (TOTAL BODY)

Exercise #1: Knees to Elbows	11 reps
Exercise #2: Dive Bombers	7 reps
Exercise #3: Mountain Climbers	11 reps

The Enduro Mission

This strategy's all about maximum repetitions. The Missions challenge and develop your muscular and cardiorespiratory endurance and your stamina. Three minutes is a long time when you're performing a single exercise. You can expect to build up a big burn in your muscles and hit a wall that stops you from performing any more reps. When you reach that wall, simply use the +2 method and continue chipping away at your reps until you finish the 3-minute interval!

Goal: *Do as many repetitions as possible during each 3-minute interval.*

Breakthrough Training Tactic: *+2 method*

What You'll Need: *a stopwatch, a clock with a sweeping hand, or a smartphone app with timer*

PROTOCOL

1. Do as many Exercise #1 repetitions as you can in 3 minutes.
2. Immediately do as many Exercise #2 repetitions as you can in 3 minutes.
3. Immediately do as many Exercise #3 repetitions as you can in 3 minutes.

Right on! 3 exercises for 3 minutes each = a 9-Minute Mission!

Four Great Enduro Missions

(See the 9-Minute Mission exercise instructions following the five Mission protocols for information on these exercises.)

PUSH 'N' PRESS (UPPER BODY)
   Exercise #1: Triangle Push-Ups
   Exercise #2: Bench Dip
   Exercise #3: Pike Press

BUTT OUT (LOWER BODY)
   Exercise #1: Squat Jacks
   Exercise #2: Marching Soldiers
   Exercise #3: Back Lunge

THE WASHBOARD (CORE)
   Exercise #1: Mountain Climbers
   Exercise #2: Swing-Ups
   Exercise #3: Plank

MONDAY FUNDAY (TOTAL BODY)
   Exercise #1: Triangle Push-Ups
   Exercise #2: Twisters
   Exercise #3: Air Squats

The Stepladder Mission

This strategy's all about stepping it up. The early rounds seem easy at first, but beware: These missions sneak up on you! As the number of reps gets higher and higher with each round, you'll feel your muscles burning and your heart beating hard. Be sure to power breathe early to break through your mental barrier and beat your mission!

Goal: *Do as many circuits as possible in 9 minutes. Go as high as you can!*

Breakthrough Training Tactic: *power breathing*

What You'll Need: *a stopwatch, a clock with a sweeping hand, or a smartphone app with timer.*

PROTOCOL

1. Do 1 circuit of 1 repetition of each of the 3 exercises.
2. Do 1 circuit of 2 repetitions of each exercise.
3. Ladder up: Do a 3-rep circuit, then a 4-rep circuit, etc., to complete as many circuits as you can in 9 minutes.

Check it out: 9 minutes of laddering up = a 9-Minute Mission!

Four Great Stepladder Missions

(See the 9-Minute Mission exercise instructions following the five Mission protocols for information on these exercises.)

HARD CORE (CORE)
Exercise #1: Swing-Ups
Exercise #2: Knees to Elbows
Exercise #3: Mountain Climbers

THE PULSE POUNDER (TOTAL BODY)
Exercise #1: Burpee
Exercise #2: Knees to Elbows
Exercise #3: Air Squat

DRILL SERGEANT (UPPER BODY)
Exercise #1: Commander Push-Ups
Exercise #2: Pike Press
Exercise #3: Burpee

STEP IT UP (LOWER BODY)

    Exercise #1: Back Lunge

    Exercise #2: Bridge-Ups

    Exercise #3: Squat Jacks

The Super Circuit Mission

This strategy's all about pacing yourself. Don't come out of the gates sprinting on this one. That's what the Rapid Rounds Missions are all about. These Missions are about finding a challenging but steady pace for doing a 3-exercise circuit over and over again for 9 minutes. Use power breathing early on in your Mission and stay focused there. Your muscles will burn and your mind will wander, but keep coming back to your breathing. Push yourself beyond your comfort zone—break through your mental barrier! You can do it!

Goal: *Complete as many circuits as possible in 9 minutes.*

Breakthrough Training Tactic: *power breathing*

What You'll Need: *a stopwatch, a clock with a sweeping hand, or a smartphone app with timer*

PROTOCOL

1. Perform the set number of repetitions of Exercise #1, immediately followed by the set number of repetitions of Exercise #2 and the set number of repetitions of Exercise #3 to complete a circuit.

2. Repeat the circuit continuously for 9 minutes.

Done! 9 minutes of continuous circuits = a 9-Minute Mission!

Four Great Super Circuit Missions

(See the 9-Minute Mission exercise instructions following the five Mission protocols for information on these exercises.)

STACK 'EM UP (TOTAL BODY)

Exercise #1: Squat Thrusts	5 reps
Exercise #2: Swing-Ups	10 reps
Exercise #3: Marching Soldiers	15 reps

CRAZY EIGHTS (UPPER BODY)

Exercise #1: Mountain Climber	8 reps
Exercise #2: Bench Dip	8 reps
Exercise #3: Dive Bomber	8 reps

DROP IT LIKE IT'S HOT (LOWER BODY)

Exercise #1: High Knees	30 reps
Exercise #2: Back Lunge	20 reps
Exercise #3: Squat Jacks	10 reps

LUCKY THIRTEEN (CORE)

Exercise #1: Swing-Ups	13 reps
Exercise #2: Mountain Climbers	13 reps
Exercise #3: Twisters	13 reps

Your 9-Minute Mission Exercises

Your body is made to run, jump, push, pull, crunch, and squat. This is how we move through life! We squat when getting in and out of a car, we crunch when we sit up in bed, we push up when getting off of the ground, we run when we need to get somewhere quickly. Every exercise in the 9-Minute Missions incorporates these fundamental movements of the human body. In essence, by doing your 9-Minute Missions you're training for real life.

With thirty exercises to choose from, I really mix it up in the twenty 9-Minute Missions. Whatever your mood, your energy level, or your appetite for something new, you get a brand-new mission each and every weekday for a month!

Have fun!

9-Minute Missions Terminology

Core: The muscles of the abdomen (*transversus abdominus, rectus abdominus*, internal and external obliques, and all stabilizing, supporting muscles surrounding them).

Crunch: Flexing the spine, bending forward.

Extend: Opening a joint to its fullest potential.

Lock: Holding a set joint position.

Pike position: The triangle position like the "downward dog" pose in yoga. Arms are fully extended with head tucked between the shoulders. Hips are as high in the air as possible, with legs extended and toes on the ground. Push the heels toward the floor.

Plank position: There are two variations: One is identical to the top of a push-up, rigid from heel to shoulder, with hands underneath shoulders and elbows extended. The second plank position is similar, except the body is resting on the elbows.

Warming Up and Cooling Down

Whenever you embark on your 9-Minute Mission, it is always good to warm up before you start and cool down when you're done.

Warm up fast by moving the biggest muscle groups in your body (in your legs). This increases your body temperature and the blood flow to your muscles and joints. You often do this by mimicking jumping rope or jogging in place, but you can do high knees, jumping jacks, or anything that gets your heart pumping and increases your body temperature! Then move on to 4 simple movements for 1 minute each that gently stretch and contract your muscles. The key is to keep moving through the warm-up movements and never hold any one position. You may go back and forth through the movement 6 to 8 times in the minute. This prepares your muscles to contract and relax faster, improves joint mobility, and helps to prevent injuries. Five to 6 minutes of movement makes an ideal warm-up or cool-down, but you'll benefit even from only 2 minutes if you are crunched for time. Your body's warm when you begin to break a light sweat.

Cooling down lets your heartbeat and breathing slow down gently, and prevents your blood from pooling in your extremities. You can simply walk or jog in place for a minute or two, then go through the same movements as the warm-up. Instead of continuously moving through the motions as in the warm-up, hold each position for 30 seconds during the cool-down. This is a great time to gently stretch and lengthen the muscles while they are warm.

Warm-Up Exercises

Jump rope or jog in place for 2 minutes before doing any of these exercises.

TWISTERS

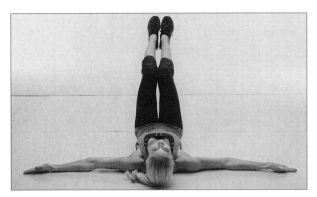

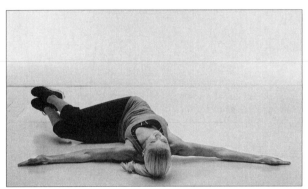

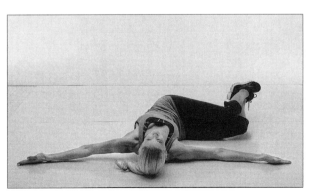

WARM UP

1 minute back and forth
in a continuous motion

COOL DOWN

hold 30 seconds
each side

SCORPIONS

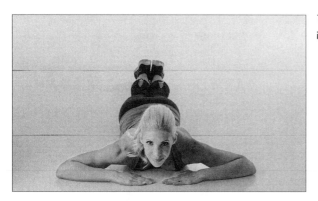

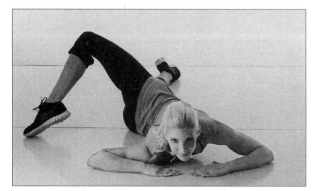

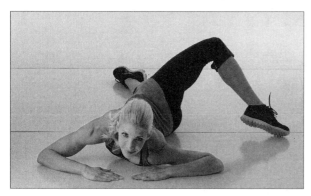

WARM UP

1 minute back and forth in a continuous motion

COOL DOWN

hold 30 seconds each side

SWOOPS

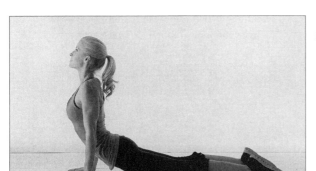

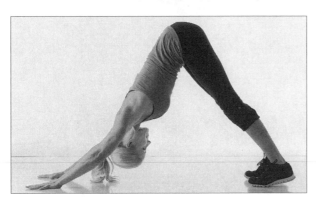

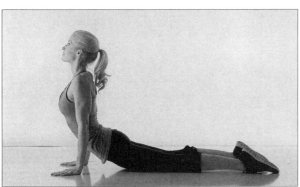

WARM UP

1 minute back and forth
in a continuous motion

COOL DOWN

hold 30 seconds
each side

DEEP LUNGE

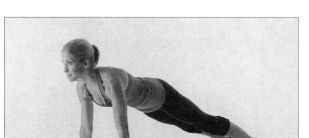

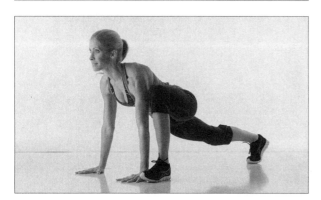

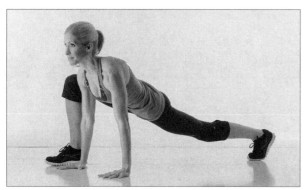

WARM UP

1 minute back and forth
in a continuous motion

COOL DOWN

hold 30 seconds
each side

Pushing (Upper Body) Exercises

Excellent for development of the chest, shoulder, and tricep muscles.

PUSH-UPS

Beginner

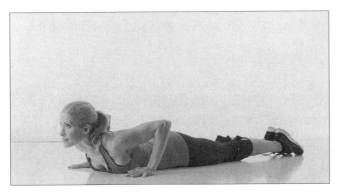

Start lying facedown on the floor, with your elbows bent and your hands on the floor beneath your shoulders.

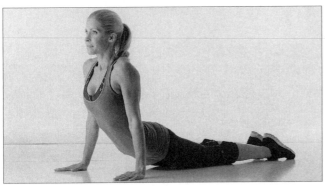

Keeping your hips on the floor, slowly press upward with your arms, extending your elbows and back.

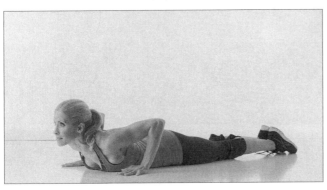

Bending your elbows, slowly lower your upper body back to the floor into the starting position.

Intermediate

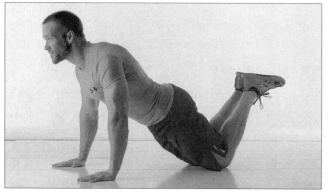

Start in the plank position with your knees together on the floor, your hands on the floor below your shoulders, and your elbows extended so you're pushed up at the shoulders. Your body should be rigid from your knees to your shoulders; your abs should be tight, and your legs should be bent up behind you at an angle of about 90 degrees. Your feet should be together.

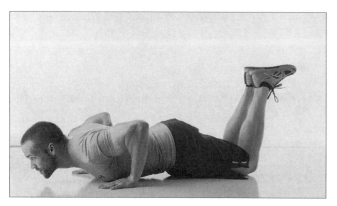

Bending your elbows, lower your body and touch your chest and thighs to the floor while staying rigid from your knees to your shoulders. Your knees should remain bent and your feet should be together in the air behind you.

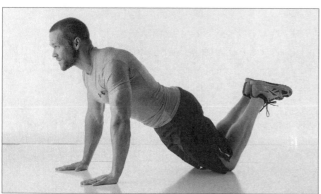

Immediately press upward again until your elbows are fully extended and you're in the starting position.

Advanced

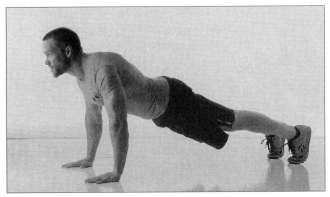

Start in the plank position with your hands on the floor below your shoulders and your elbows extended so you're pushed up at the shoulders. Your abs should be tight, and your body should be rigid from your heels to your shoulders.

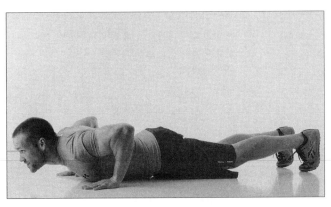

Bending your elbows, lower your body and touch your chest and thighs to the floor while staying rigid from your heels to your shoulders.

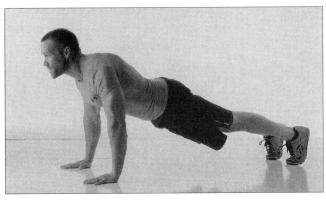

Immediately press upward again until your elbows are fully extended and you're back in the starting position.

Super-Advanced (Palm-Release Push-Ups)

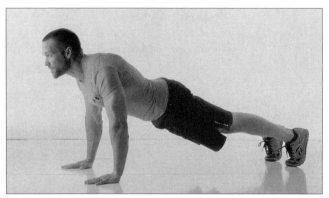

Start in the plank position with your hands on the floor below your shoulders and your elbows extended so you're pushed up at the shoulders. Your abs should be tight and body should be rigid from your heels to your shoulders.

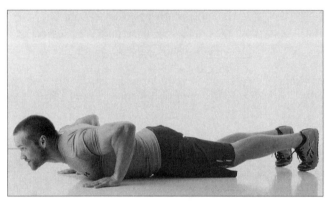

Bending your elbows, lower your body and touch your chest and thighs to the floor while staying rigid from your heels to your shoulders.

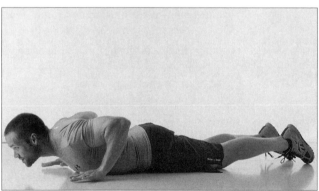

As your chest and thighs touch the floor, raise your hands a fraction of an inch off of the ground, enough so that you can slide a piece of paper underneath them.

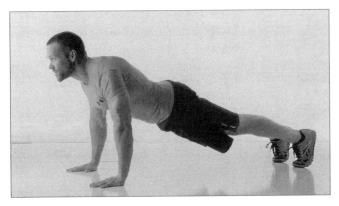

Immediately press upward again until your elbows are fully extended and you're back in the starting position.

COMMANDER PUSH-UPS

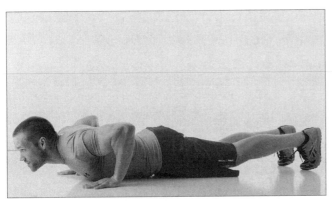

Start lying facedown on the floor, with your hands aligned beneath your shoulders, your abs tight, and your body rigid.

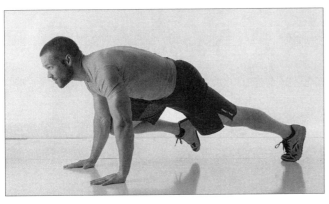

Press upward, extending your elbows while driving your right knee forward and touching it to your right elbow.

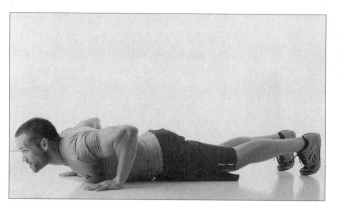

Extending your right leg behind you again, bend your elbows and lower your body to the floor, staying rigid from your feet to your shoulders.

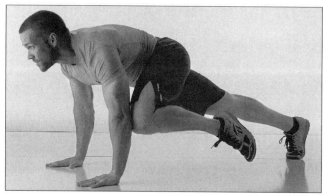

Press upward again, extending your elbows while driving your left knee forward and touching it to your left elbow.

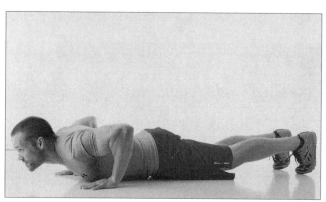

Return to the starting position by extending your left leg behind you, bending your elbows, and lowering your body to the floor, staying rigid from your feet to your shoulders.

TRIANGLE PUSH-UPS

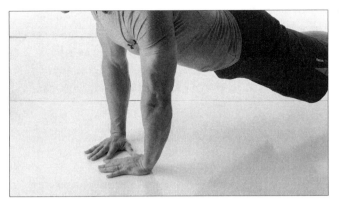

This movement is identical to the standard push-up, except your hands should be positioned to create a triangle between your index fingers and thumbs.

DIVE BOMBERS

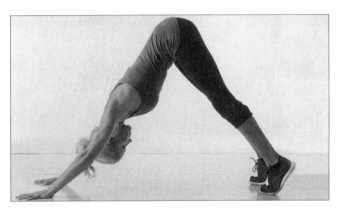

Start in the pike position, bent over in a V at the waist with your hips high in the air, your hands and toes on the floor, and your elbows and knees extended. The angle between your torso and legs should be slightly less than 90 degrees, and your head and neck should be straight.

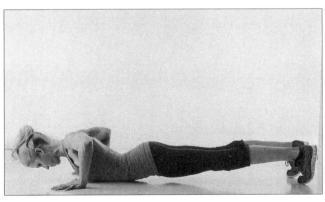

Bending your elbows, shift your weight forward, lowering your chest and thighs to the floor while straightening out your body.

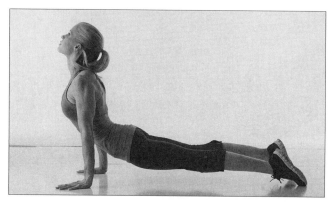

While pressing upward again, swing your body forward, arch your back, and bring your head forward and up in a swooping movement, passing it through the air just above your hands. Extend your elbows and knees and keep your body suspended between your shoulders and your toes.

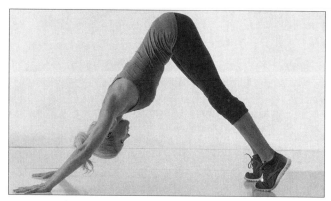

Shift your body back to the pike position again and prepare for another dive bomber!

BENCH DIP

Beginner

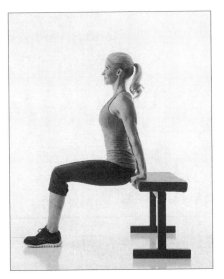

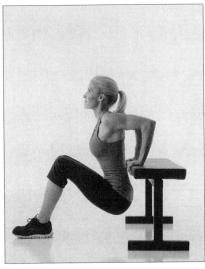

Start in a seated position with your knees bent at 90 degrees and your hips held a couple of inches in front of a seat, at seat level. Support yourself with your hands behind you on the seat, with your elbows extended. Your hands should be spaced shoulder-width apart.

Lower your body, bending your elbows to a 90-degree angle.

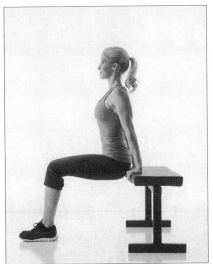

Press upward through your palms until your elbows are fully extended, your hips are at seat level, and you're in the starting position.

Advanced

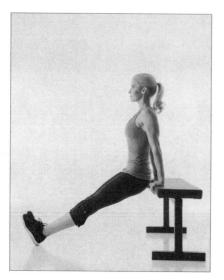

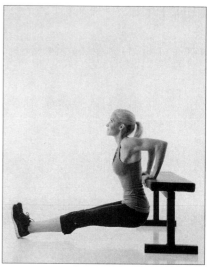

Start in a seated position with your knees extended and locked, your heels on the floor, and your hips held a couple of inches in front of a seat, at seat level. Support yourself with your hands behind you on the seat, with your elbows extended. Your hands should be spaced apart at shoulder width.

Lower your body, bending your elbows to a 90-degree angle.

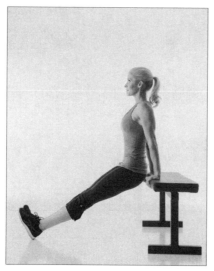

Press upward through your palms until your elbows are fully extended, your hips are at seat level, and you're in the starting position.

PIKE PRESS

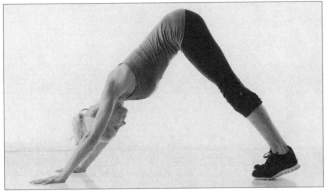

Start in the pike position, bent over in a V at the waist with your hips high in the air, your hands and the balls of your feet on the floor, and your elbows and knees extended. The angle between your torso and legs should be slightly less than 90 degrees, and your head and neck should be straight.

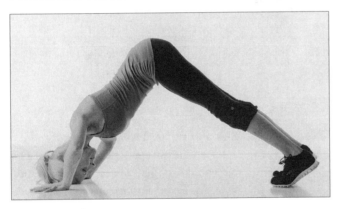

Bending at the elbows, lower your head to the floor until your forehead touches it.

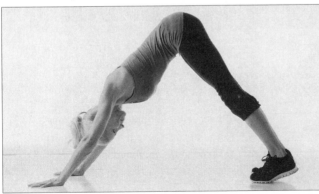

Press up and backward to the starting position.

Crunching (Core) Exercises

Excellent for core strength, midline stability, and development of the abs and lower back.

SWING-UPS

Beginner

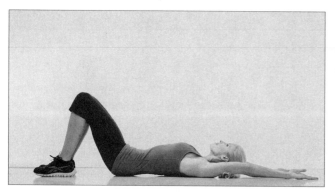

Start lying faceup on the floor with your knees bent, your feet flat on the floor, and your arms extended overhead and resting on the floor.

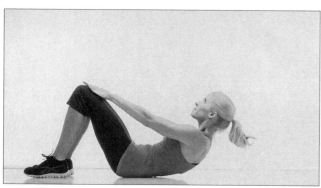

Swing your arms up and forward in an arc over and past your head, using the momentum to raise your shoulders off the floor. Keeping your back straight and your elbows extended, touch the palms of your hands to the tops of your knees.

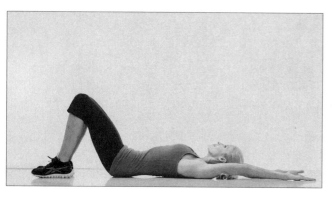

Reverse the motion and lower your shoulders back to the floor with arms overhead to starting position.

Intermediate

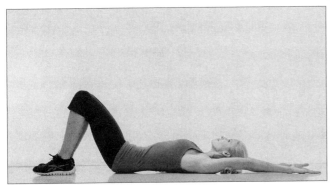

Start lying faceup on the floor with your knees bent, your feet flat on the floor, and your arms extended overhead and resting on the floor.

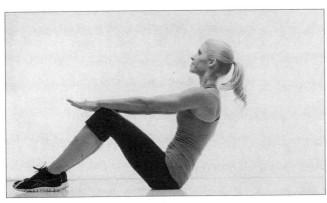

Swing your arms up and forward in an arc over and past your head, using the momentum to raise your shoulders and torso off the floor. Keeping your back straight and your elbows extended, touch your wrists to the tops of your knees.

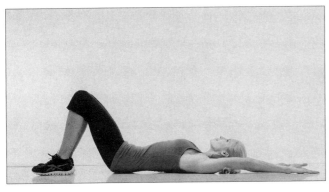

Keeping your elbows extended, reverse the motion as you lower your torso and shoulders back to the floor, with arms extended overhead.

Advanced

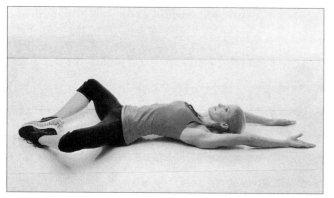

Start lying faceup on the floor with the bottoms of your feet touching and your knees bent and dropped to the side in a "butterfly" position. Extend your arms overhead so they are resting on the floor.

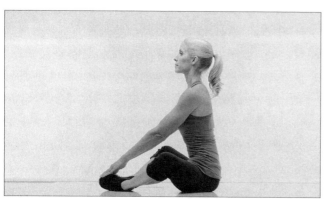

Swing your arms up and forward in an arc over and past your head, using the momentum to raise your shoulders and torso off the floor. Keeping your back straight and your elbows extended, touch your toes with your fingertips.

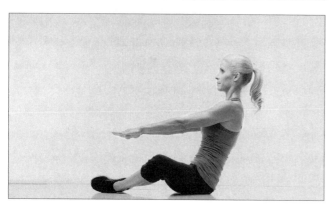

Keeping your elbows extended, reverse the motion as you lower your torso and shoulders back to the floor.

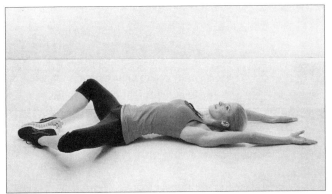

With your arms overhead in the starting position, touch the floor with the backs of your hands.

PLANK

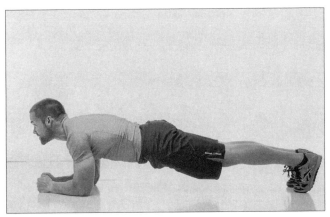

Start in a facedown position, propped up on your elbows, with your elbows aligned directly beneath your shoulders and your forearms resting on the floor. Your knees should be fully extended and your toes on the floor. Squeeze your glutes, draw your belly button in toward your spine and raise your hips approximately one foot above the floor. Your body should be rigid and elevated from heels to shoulders. Hold the position as long as you can. Lower hips to the ground when you need to rest.

TWISTERS

Beginner

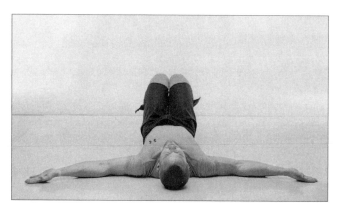

Start lying faceup on the floor, with your knees bent, your feet flat on the floor, and your arms extended outward like wings resting on the floor.

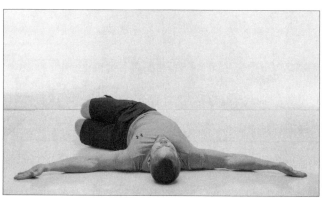

Keeping your shoulders and arms anchored to the floor and your knees together, tilt your knees over to your left side. Touch your left knee to the floor to mark a complete repetition.

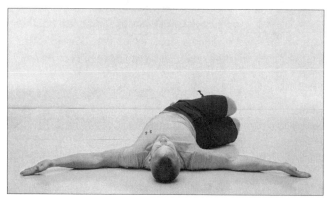

Keeping your shoulders and arms anchored to the floor and your knees together, bring your knees 180 degrees over to your right side. Touch your right knee to the floor to mark another repetition. Return your legs to the starting position.

Intermediate

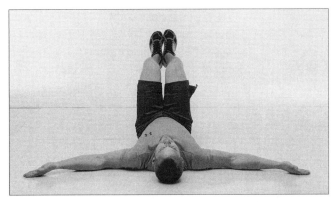

Start lying faceup on the floor, holding your thighs in the air perpendicular to the floor and your knees bent at a 90-degree angle, as if you're sitting in an overturned chair. Your knees should be together and your arms extended outward like wings resting on the floor.

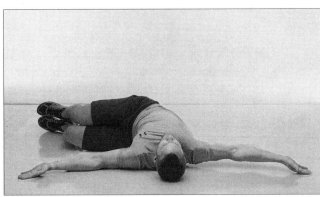

Keeping your legs in their "sitting" formation, your shoulders and arms anchored to the floor, and your knees together, tip your legs over to your left side. Touch your left knee to the floor to mark a complete repetition.

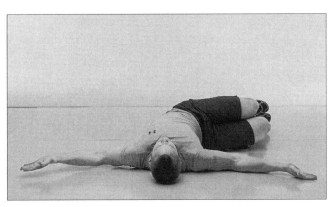

Keeping your legs in their "sitting" forma-tion, your shoulders and arms anchored to the floor, and your knees together, bring your knees 180 degrees over to your right side. Touch your right knee to the floor to mark another repetition. Return your legs to the starting position.

Advanced

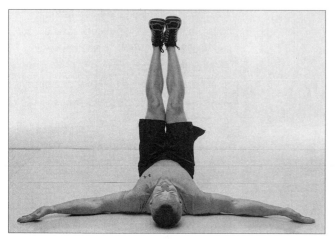

Start lying faceup on the floor, holding your legs in the air perpendicular to the floor, your legs straight, and your arms extended outward like wings resting on the floor.

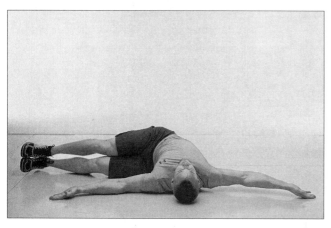

Keeping your shoulders and arms anchored to the floor and your legs together, swing your legs over to your left side. Touch your left foot to the floor to mark a complete repetition.

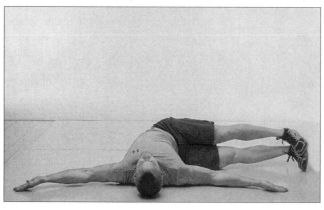

Keeping your shoulders and arms anchored to the floor and your legs together, bring your legs 180 degrees over to your right side. Touch your right foot to the floor to mark another repetition. Return your legs to the starting position.

KNEES TO ELBOWS

Beginner

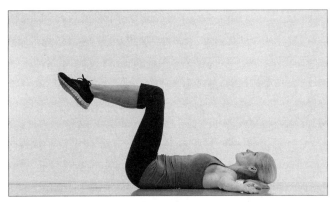

Start lying faceup on the floor with your knees and hips bent at a 90-degree angle, like sitting in a chair, arms extended out to the sides.

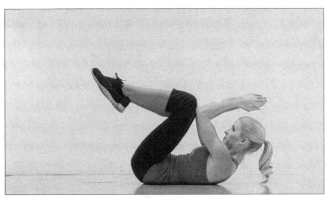

In one movement, draw your knees slightly toward your chest, bringing your elbows in to touch your knees, crunching upward with your torso so your buttocks and shoulders lift off the floor.

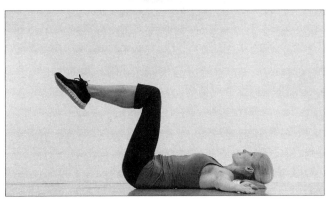

Bring your legs back to the "chair" position, lowering your torso back to the floor, and extend your arms out to the sides.

Advanced

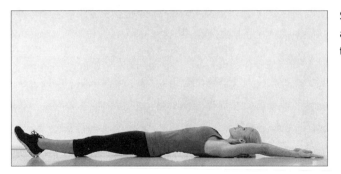

Start lying faceup on the floor with your arms extended overhead, hands and heels touching the floor.

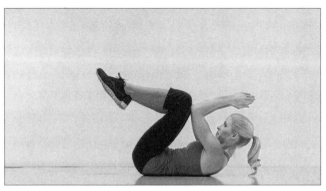

In one movement, draw your knees up toward your chest and your elbows down toward your hips, crunching upward with your torso so your buttocks and shoulders lift off the floor. Touch your elbows to your knees.

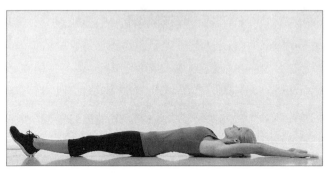

Extend your legs all the way back downward and your arms all the way back overhead. Touch your heels and the backs of your hands to the floor, returning to the starting position.

Squatting (Lower Body) Exercises

Excellent for development of the glutes (butt), quads, and hamstrings (thighs).

AIR SQUATS

Beginner

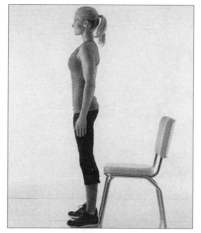

Start by standing in front of a chair, facing away from the chair. Your feet should be shoulder-width apart, your toes pointed slightly outward and your hips and knees fully extended.

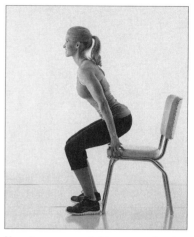

Keeping your weight on your heels, slowly lower your hips onto the seat of the chair, as if you're being pulled backward by your belt. Reach backward with your hands to help guide you.

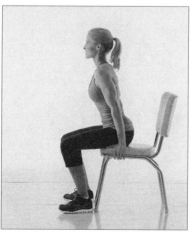

Sit on the chair and allow the weight in your hips to shift backward, as you would when sitting normally.

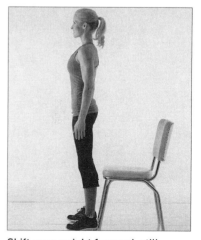

Shift your weight forward, still keeping your weight on your heels, and stand up to the starting position, with your knees and hips extended. Use your hands to push off of the chair if needed.

Intermediate

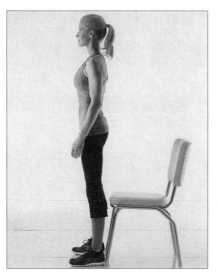

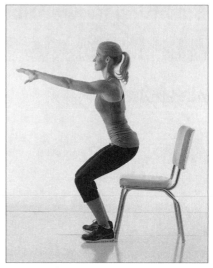

Start by standing in front of a chair, facing away from the chair. Your feet should be shoulder-width apart, your toes pointed slightly outward and your hips and knees fully extended.

Keeping your weight on your heels, slowly lower your hips onto the seat of the chair, as if you're being pulled backward by your belt.

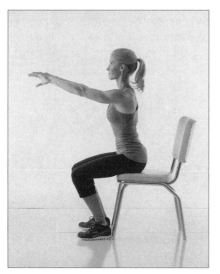

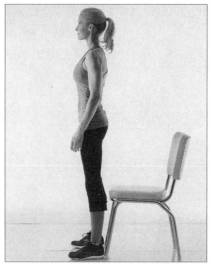

Extend your arms in front of you, using them as a counterbalance, and gently touch the seat with your hips, making sure that your knees are tracking directly over your toes and not knocking inward.

As soon as you feel your hips touch the seat, drive upward through your heels, fully extending your knees and hips to stand up to the starting position.

Advanced

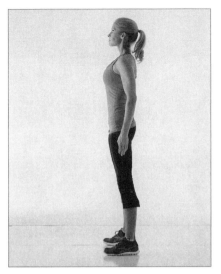

Start by standing with your feet shoulder-width apart, your toes pointed slightly outward, and your hips and knees fully extended.

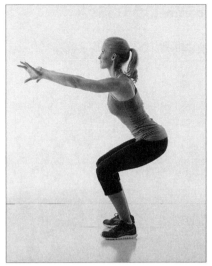

Keeping your weight on your heels, bend your knees and lower your hips down and back, as if you're being pulled backward by your belt.

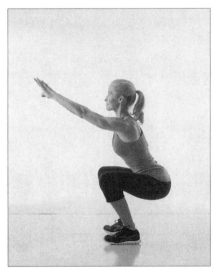

Using your arms as a counterbalance, reach upward as your hips drop slightly below your knees. Make sure that your knees are tracking directly over your toes and not knocking inward.

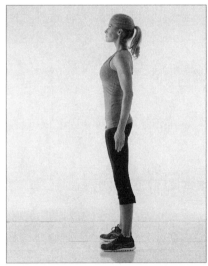

Drive upward through your heels, fully extending your knees and hips to stand up to the starting position.

BACK LUNGES

Beginner

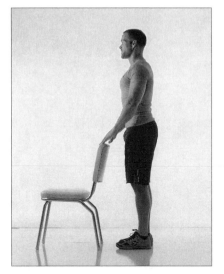

Start by standing with your hips and knees fully extended, holding onto a chair or other stable object.

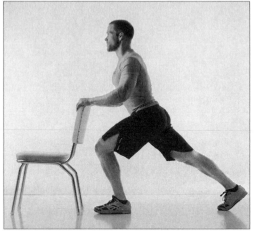

Take an aggressive step backward with your right foot, fully extending that leg and touching the floor with the toes of that foot. Allow your left knee to bend and your body to lower slightly to adjust for the movement.

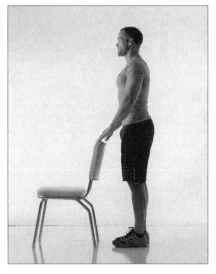

Keeping your left knee directly over the toes of your left foot, drive through your left heel and draw your right leg forward to bring your body to a standing position.

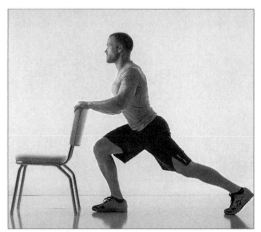

Take an aggressive step backward with your left foot, fully extending that leg and touching the floor with the toes of that foot. Allow your right knee to bend and your body to lower slightly to adjust for the movement.

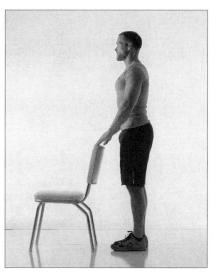

Keeping your right knee directly over the toes of your right foot, drive through your right heel and draw your left leg forward to bring your body to the starting position.

Intermediate

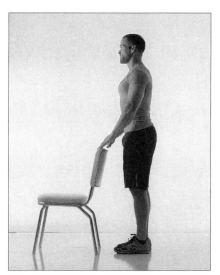

Start by standing with your hips and knees fully extended, holding onto a chair or other stable object.

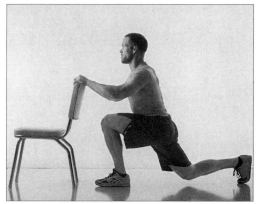

Take an aggressive step backward with your right foot and gently "kiss" the floor with your right knee. Bend your left knee to adjust for the movement.

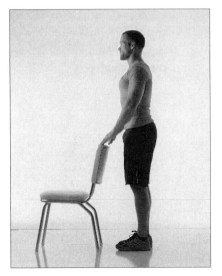

Keeping your left knee directly over the toes of your left foot, drive through your left heel and draw your right leg forward to bring your body to a standing position.

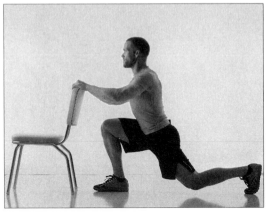

Take an aggressive step backward with your left foot and gently "kiss" the floor with your left knee. Bend your right knee to adjust for the movement.

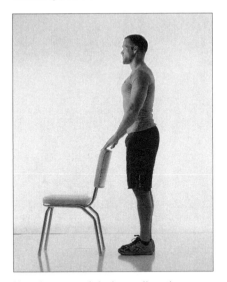

Keeping your right knee directly over the toes of your right foot, drive through your right heel and draw your left leg forward to bring your body to the starting position.

Advanced

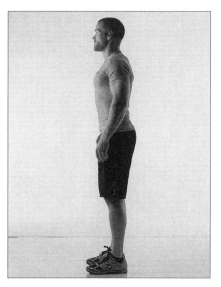

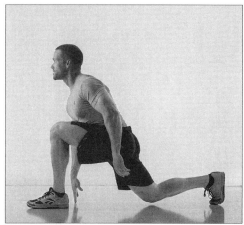

Start by standing with your hips and knees fully extended and your arms relaxed at your sides.

Take an aggressive step backward with your right foot, gently "kiss" the floor with your right knee, and touch the floor with your right hand. Bend your left knee to adjust for the movement.

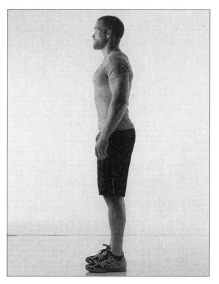

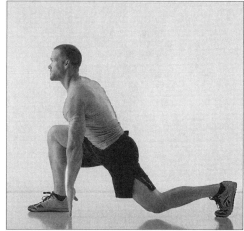

Keeping your left knee directly over the toes of your left foot, drive through your left heel and draw your right leg forward to bring your body to a standing position.

Take an aggressive step backward with your left foot, gently "kiss" the floor with your left knee, and touch the floor with your left hand. Bend your right knee to adjust for the movement.

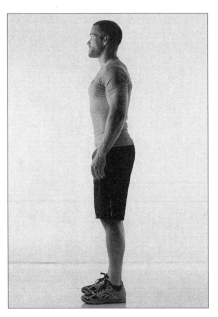

Keeping your right knee directly over the toes of your right foot, drive through your right heel and draw your left leg forward to bring your body to the starting position.

BRIDGE-UPS

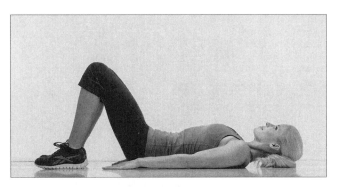

Start lying faceup on the floor with your knees bent, your feet flat on the floor, and your arms relaxed at your sides.

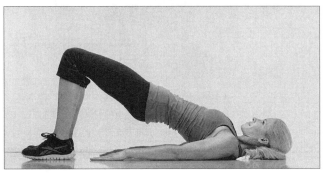

Squeeze your glutes to press your lower back into the floor, then raise your hips off the floor as high as you can, pressing through your heels. Keep your arms anchored to the floor.

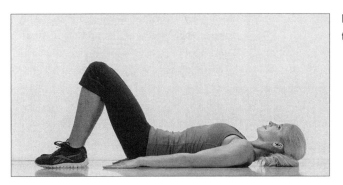

Lower your hips back to the floor and return to the starting position.

MARCHING SOLDIERS

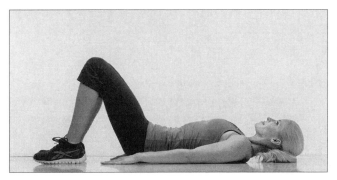

Start lying faceup on the floor with your knees bent, your feet flat on the floor, and your arms relaxed at your sides.

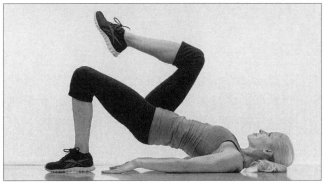

Driving your left heel into the floor, raise your hips as high as you can and keep your right knee bent while lifting it as far as you can toward your chest.

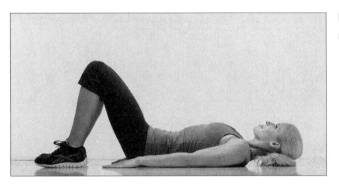

Lower your right leg back to the floor and return to the starting position.

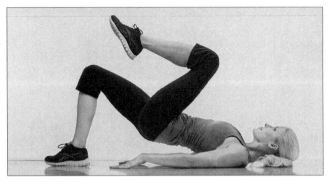

Quickly switch sides and drive your right heel into the floor, raising your hips again. Keep your left knee bent while lifting it as far as you can toward your chest.

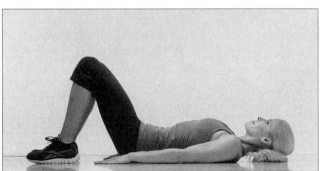

Lower your left leg and hips back to the floor and return to the starting position.

Running and Jumping (Total Body) Exercises

Excellent for the development of multiple muscle systems.

HIGH KNEES

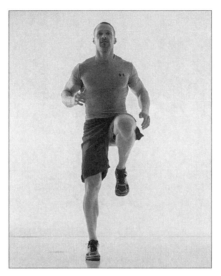 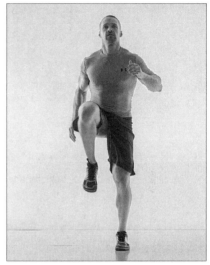

Keeping your weight on your toes, run in place, bringing your knees up toward your chest as high as you can. With your elbows at a 90-degree angle, pump your arms aggressively at your sides, in time with your running movement.

JOGGING IN PLACE

Beginner version of High Knees

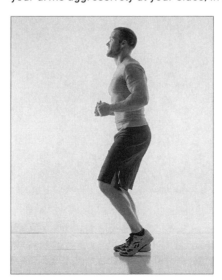 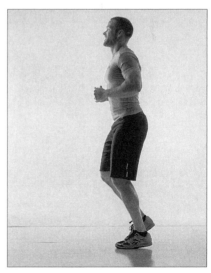

Bending your arms at a 90-degree angle, begin jogging in place by raising one heel after the other with a slight spring in your step. To keep this movement low-impact, keep toes on the ground and simply raise heels as you jog in place.

RUNNING IN PLACE

Intermediate version of High Knees

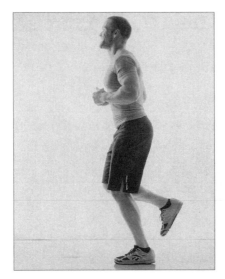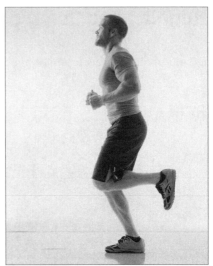

Run in place, kicking your legs back, keeping your elbows at a 90-degree angle and pumping your arms at your sides in time with your running movement.

SQUAT JACKS

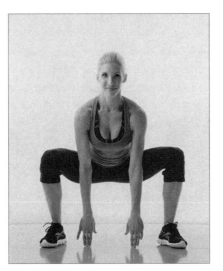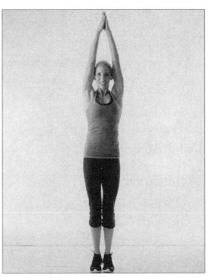

Start by squatting with your feet and knees wide apart and your hips a few inches lower than your knees. Lean forward with your back flat and your eyes aimed directly ahead, your arms extended straight down from your shoulders (between your legs), and your fingertips touching the floor.

In one quick movement, jump up, fully extend your legs, bring your feet together, and fully extend your arms overhead to clap your hands.

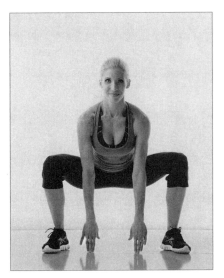

Jump your feet back out to a wide stance and quickly drop back into a squat, touching the floor with your fingertips to return to the starting position.

STEP JACKS

Beginner version of Squat Jacks

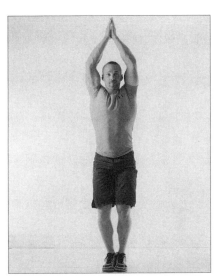

Start by standing with your feet together, your legs and back straight, your shoulders squared, your arms fully extended up overhead.

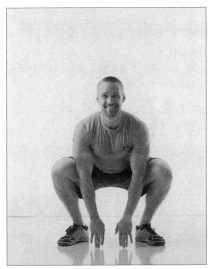

Step to the side, squatting downward and touching the ground. Be sure to keep your chest up and drop your hips as low as you can.

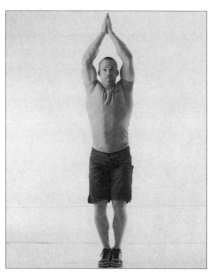

Extend upward, bringing your feet back together and clapping your hands overhead.

JUMPING JACKS

Intermediate version of Squat Jacks

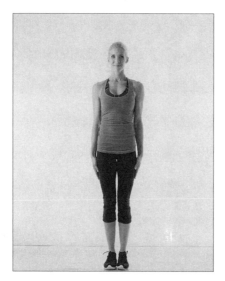

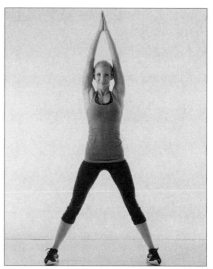

Start by standing with your feet together, your legs and back straight, your shoulders squared, your arms fully extended down from your shoulders, and your hands at your sides.

In one quick movement, jump your feet out to a wide stance, keeping your knees fully extended. Swing your arms out from your sides and up over your head to point straight upward and clap your hands.

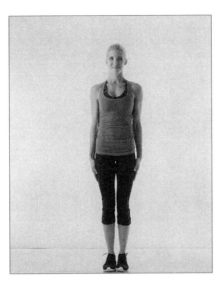

Jump your feet back together and bring your arms quickly back down to your sides, returning to the starting position.

JUMP ROPE

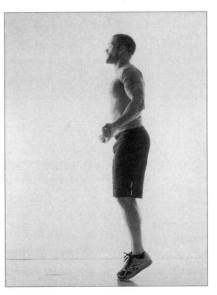

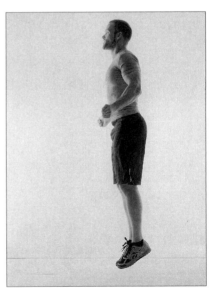

Grab a jump rope or just pretend you have one! Standing tall with your chest out, spring off of the ground 1 to 3 inches with each hop.

Be sure to stay rigid through the core and extend the hips and ankles fully with each jump.

BURPEE

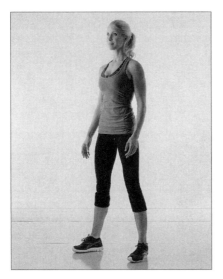 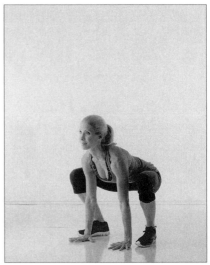

Start by standing with your feet shoulder-width apart, your toes pointed slightly outward, your back straight, and your hands hanging loosely at your sides.

Assume a frog-squat position by bending your knees and lowering your body until your hips are a few inches lower than your knees. Lean forward with your back flat and your eyes aimed directly ahead, until your shoulders are a few inches higher than your knees. Extend your arms straight down from your shoulders (between your legs) and place your hands flat on the floor.

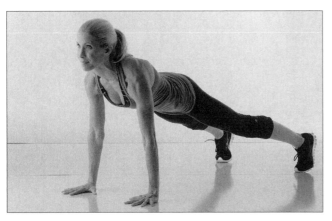

Keeping your hands on the floor at shoulder width and bracing yourself on your fully extended arms, jump or walk your feet backward and land on your toes, with your feet shoulder-width apart. Finish the movement in the plank position, rigid from your shoulders to your heels and supporting yourself on your hands and toes.

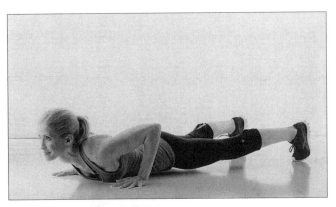

Bending your elbows, lower your body to the floor.

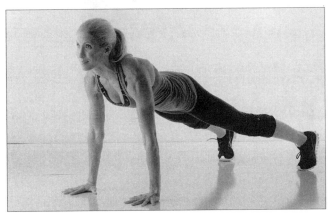

Perform a push-up by fully extending your elbows and straightening your arms, finishing in the plank position.

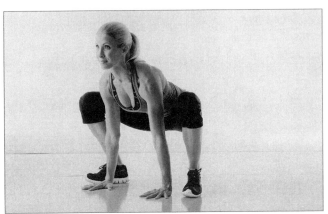

Jump or walk your feet forward to assume the frog-squat position.

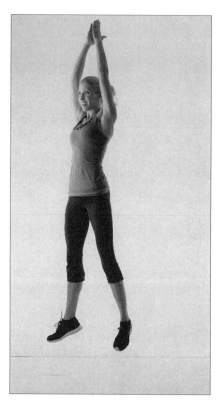

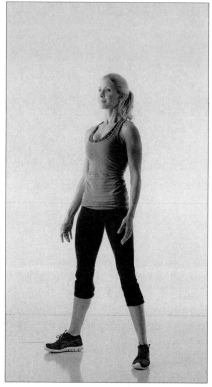

Jump upward into the air in one movement, extending your knees and straightening your legs. Swing your arms out from your sides and up over your head to point straight upward and clap your hands.

Land in the starting position.

SQUAT THRUSTS

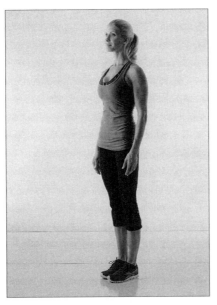

Start by standing with your feet and knees together, your back straight, and your hands hanging loosely at your sides.

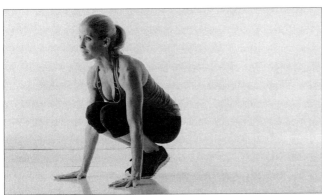

Keeping your back straight and your feet and knees together, go into a squatting position by bending your knees and lowering your hips toward the floor. Drop your hips until they are several inches lower than your knees and your chest touches the tops of your thighs. Place your hands on the floor shoulder-width apart, with your arms straight and outside your knees.

Supporting yourself on your hands, thrust your feet back.

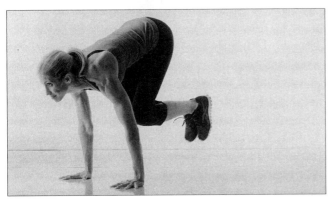

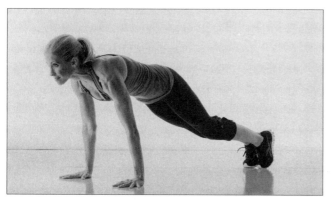

Straightening your knees, land in the plank position with your abs tight and your body rigid from heels to shoulders. Only your hands and toes should be touching the floor, and your elbows should be fully extended.

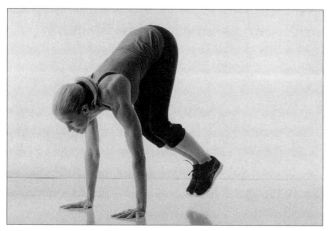

Jump your feet forward.

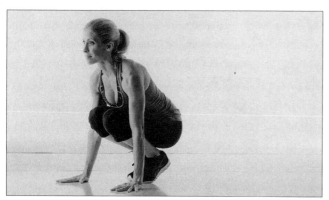

Land in the squatting position.

Stand up, fully extending your knees and hips to end in the starting position.

DOWN AND UPS

Beginner version of Burpee and Squat Thrusts

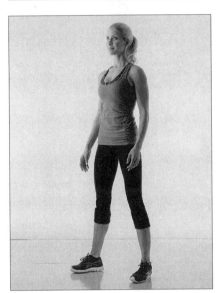

Start by standing with your feet shoulder-width apart, your toes pointed slightly outward, your back straight, and your hands hanging loosely at your sides.

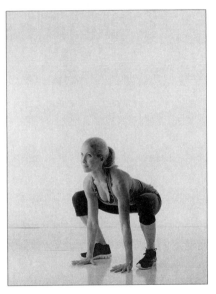

Assume a frog-squat position by bending your knees and lowering your body until your hips are a few inches lower than your knees. Lean forward with your back flat and your eyes aimed directly ahead, until your shoulders are a few inches higher than your knees. Extend your arms straight down from your shoulders (between your legs) and place your hands flat on the floor.

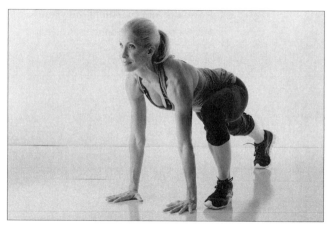

Extend your right leg out behind you. If this is too difficult, you may place your right knee on the ground.

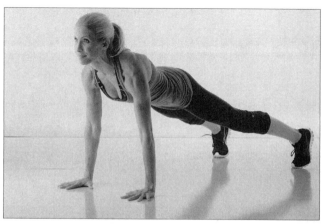

Extend your left leg out behind you to a plank position. If this is too difficult, you may place your left knee on the ground.

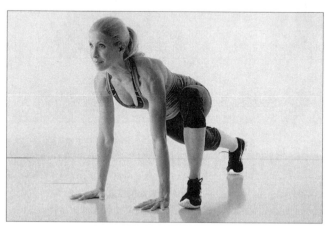

Step forward with your left foot, placing it just outside and behind your left hand.

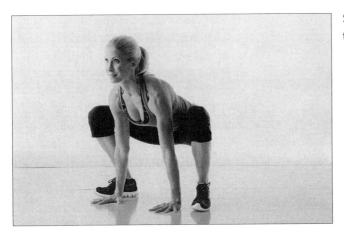

Step forward with your right foot, returning to the frog-squat position.

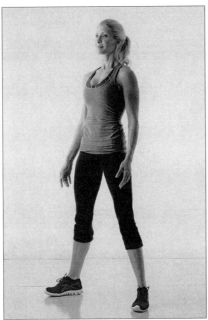

Stand up, driving through your heels to reach the starting position.

MOUNTAIN CLIMBERS

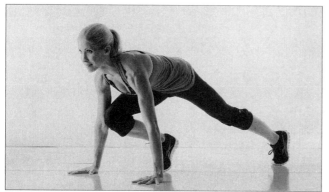

Start in a deep runner's starting stance, with both hands on the floor at shoulder width, your right knee thrust forward to just inside your right elbow and your left leg extended all the way behind you. You should be on your toes, with your back and arms straight and your eyes looking directly to the front.

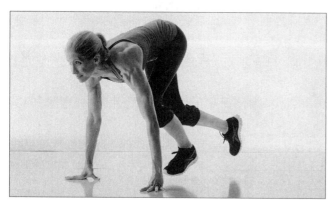

Supporting yourself on your hands and keeping your abs tight, jump to switch the positions of your feet as fast as you can.

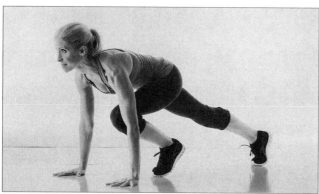

Land gently in the starting position, but with your left knee forward and your right leg extended back.

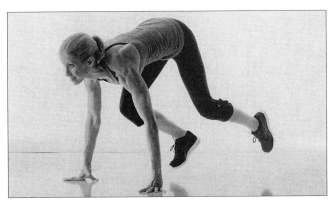

As soon as your feet touch down, jump to switch the positions of your feet again.

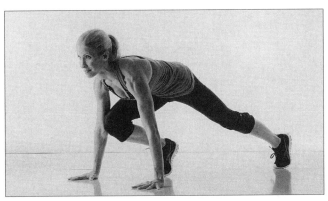

Land gently in the starting position, with your right knee forward and your left leg extended back.

WALKING THE PLANK

Intermediate version of Mountain Climbers

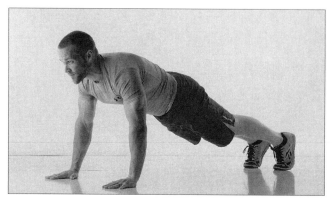

Start in the plank position with your toes a few inches apart on the floor, your hands on the floor below your shoulders and your elbows extended so you're pushed up at the shoulders. Your body should be rigid from your toes to your shoulders and your abs should be tight.

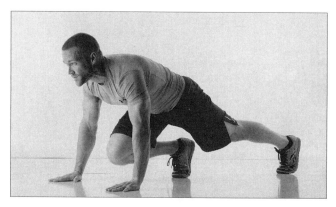

Keeping your abs tight, bring your right foot forward as far as you can and touch your toe to the floor.

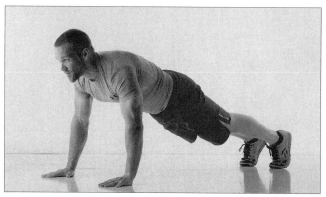

As soon as your toe touches the floor, extend your right leg behind you again so you're back in the plank position.

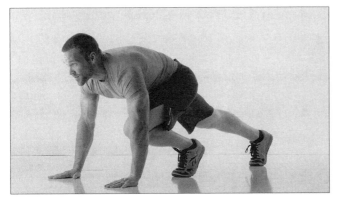

Keeping your abs tight, bring your left foot forward as far as you can and touch your toe to the floor.

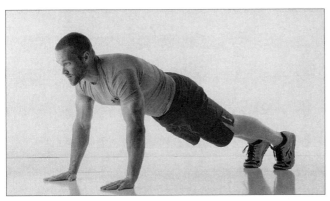

As soon as your toe touches the floor, extend your left leg behind you again so you're back in the starting position.

Your Monthly 9-Minute Mission Schedule

Okay, you've got the Sprinterval, Rapid Rounds, Enduro, Stepladder, and Super Circuit protocols for your 9-Minute Mission. You've got the thirty 9-Minute Mission exercises based on your body's basic running, jumping, pushing, squatting, and crunching movements. So how do you figure out which missions to do on which days, and how to organize them into a week or a month of workouts? You don't have to think about it, because I've set up an awesome plan for you!

Five days a week, four weeks a month, you do a 9-Minute Mission. (The other two days of the week you rest—no exercise at all!) One day you exercise your upper body (pushing), one day you exercise your core (crunching), and one day you exercise your lower body (squatting); two days a week you exercise your entire body. I've split your schedule up like this so you avoid overtraining any particular muscle. Yes, you will end up exercising certain muscles two days in a row, because your total-body workouts and your muscle-group workouts fall on adjacent days. But that's the max! After that they'll always have at least one day of rest before you exercise them again.

9 Minute Missions and Mission Types

Focus of 9 Minute Missions
Rotate between areas of focus for optimal effectiveness

Putting It All Together
Quickly identify which Mission Type you are focusing on and which body area you are working out during each 9 Minute Mission

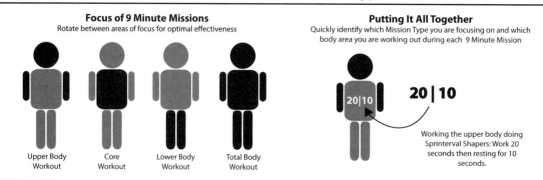

Upper Body Workout
Core Workout
Lower Body Workout
Total Body Workout

20 | 10

Working the upper body doing Sprinterval Shapers: Work 20 seconds then resting for 10 seconds.

5 Mission Types

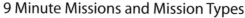

Combining 30 exercises with these 5 missions, will provide endless workouts. See exercise descriptions and Appendix for prescribed reps.

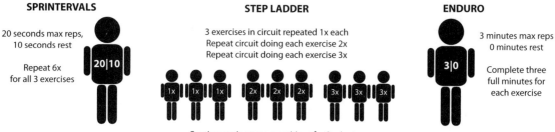

SPRINTERVALS
20 seconds max reps, 10 seconds rest

Repeat 6x for all 3 exercises

20|10

STEP LADDER
3 exercises in circuit repeated 1x each
Repeat circuit doing each exercise 2x
Repeat circuit doing each exercise 3x

1x 1x 1x   2x 2x 2x   3x 3x 3x

Continue to increase repetitions for 9 minutes

ENDURO
3 minutes max reps
0 minutes rest

3|0

Complete three full minutes for each exercise

RAPID ROUNDS
Complete as many circuits as you can of the 3 exercises, and their prescribed reps of each, in 2 minutes.
1 minute rest. Continue for 9 minutes.

 Perform complete prescribed reps for exercise 1

 Perform complete prescribed reps for exercise 2

 Perform complete prescribed reps for exercise 3

SUPER CIRCUITS
Complete as many circuits as you can of the 3 exercises, and their prescribed reps of each, in 3 minutes.
0 minutes rest. Continue for 9 minutes.

 Perform prescribed reps for exercise 1

 Perform prescribed reps for exercise 2

 Perform prescribed reps for exercise 3

To vary your 9-Minute Missions even more, I've *randomized* the order in which you use the different protocols. This means that each day you'll be exercising your muscle groups, or your total body, according to a different protocol. Each week of the month, the protocols and body zones get switched around, so no week is the same. This keeps your muscles guessing about what kind of stimulation's coming next, so they can't adapt to a routine. It'll make your fitness surge!

Here's your monthly schedule. Go for it!

9 Minute Missions - Month at a Glance

WEEK 1	Monday	Tuesday	Wednesday	Thursday	Friday	Saturday	Sunday
9-Minute Mission	Stack 'em Up	Push n' Press	Hard Core	Thigh Master	Five Alive	Rest	Rest
Mission Type:	Super Circuits	Enduro	Step Ladder	Sprinterval	Rapid Rounds		

WEEK 2	Monday	Tuesday	Wednesday	Thursday	Friday	Saturday	Sunday
9-Minute Mission	Run Like The Wind	Crazy Eights	Easy Threezies	Butt Out	The Pulse Pounder	Rest	Rest
Mission Type:	Sprintervals	Super Circuits	Rapid Rounds	Enduro	Step Ladder		

WEEK 3	Monday	Tuesday	Wednesday	Thursday	Friday	Saturday	Sunday
9-Minute Mission	Jackpot	Drill Sergeant	The Washboard	Drop It Like It's Hot	TGIF	Rest	Rest
Mission Type:	Rapid Rounds	Step Ladder	Enduro	Super Circuits	Sprintervals		

WEEK 4	Monday	Tuesday	Wednesday	Thursday	Friday	Saturday	Sunday
9-Minute Mission	Monday Funday	Shoulder Shaker	Lucky Thirteen	Step It Up	Seven Eleven	Rest	Rest
Mission Type:	Enduro	Sprintervals	Super Circuits	Step Ladder	Rapid Rounds		

Destroy Your Fat—*Fast*—with Shredders

Nutrition is the first building block of carb cycling, alternating days of high-carb and low-carb intake to continually stoke your metabolism to extreme heat. Muscle development and maintenance is the second building block, using 9-Minute Missions to keep your muscles chomping right through carbs and fat. *Accelerating calorie burn* beyond that is the third building block: cardiovascular workouts called Shredders, which melt even more fat off your body. Shredders maximize your calorie use so you incinerate 200, 400, 800—maybe even 1,000 more calories a day than you would without them! This means faster weight loss: Shredders are *accelerators*.

Shredders are *daily* workouts: You do them five days a week, on both high-carb and low-carb days. On high-carb days, you've got more fuel and more energy, so you can really attack your Shredders and send your metabolism into overdrive. On low-carb days, your body can't get its energy from carbs, so it demolishes fat!

You want to lose weight faster, right? It's something you want to do *for yourself*, so absolutely carve out Shredder time in your daily schedule. You can do your Shredders anytime—after breakfast, in the afternoon, in the evening—whatever works with your schedule. And make sure to do them five days a week!

BENEFITS OF CARDIOVASCULAR TRAINING

Shredders put your body in motion and get your heart pumping—that's what *cardiovascular* (sometimes called aerobic) exercise is. Walking, jumping rope, swimming, etc.—cardio increases your *cardiorespiratory* fitness, the performance of your body's circulatory (blood) and respiratory (breathing) systems, which supply oxygen to your muscles. The goal is to move your muscles and raise your heart rate for a prolonged period of time. With each and every muscle contraction, your body incinerates calories.

The longer you move, the more calories you burn. Shredders aren't super-quick, high-intensity workouts like 9-Minute Missions: They're longer and less intense. Longer workouts? Don't worry! To lose weight, *you don't have to run for hours* on a treadmill or chug away on an elliptical machine till your mind goes numb. I promised I'd help you get you to your weight-loss goals in the least amount of time with the least amount of effort, and I keep my promises. So I've combined two powerful training principles into one incredibly effective, efficient fat-burning workout: the Shredder.

Remember, your body's designed to adapt to absolutely anything, including exercise. When your body adapts to your workout, it'll *get less out of the exercise.* It knows the drill and goes through the motions on autopilot, without making much of an effort. To accelerate your weight loss and keep it going like lightning, you've got to play tricks on your body! Shredders do that in two ways.

UPS AND DOWNS

Trainers like me—and scientists, too—know that if you do an exercise, say stair-climbing, at a single level of intensity from start to finish, it has a lot less cardio and fat burning impact than if you vary your level of exertion during the exercise. That's why people who are serious about fitness use *interval training.* And that's why Shredders do, too. The technique is simple: You start an exercise at low intensity, kick up to high intensity for a few seconds to a minute or two, then drop back down to low intensity. And repeat. Get it? You're exercising in intervals!

By cycling through high-intensity and low-intensity action, Shredders fake your body out: It has to keep responding to *unpredictable messages,* so it can't slow down. The constant activity of an exercise such as bicycling cranks up your metabolism for all-out carbohydrate burning. And it keeps your body at that peak for a long time after your workout—this is called metabolic after-burn. Interval training makes your workout the best fat-burner it can be!

POWER SURGE

Here's something really cool, even though it's kind of a training bummer: It only takes about five to six times of doing the same workout for your body to begin to adapt to it. Five to six times! After that your body won't consume as many calories during that workout, and you'll get less fat-burning bang for your time and effort bucks. But you can sneak around this with something that I've built into Shredders: *progressive overload*. It's a tactic that steps up your cardio training every several workouts —pretty much once a week. Your Shredder workout constantly evolves, so it keeps working for you. It keeps accelerating fat loss, smashing through your weight-loss plateaus, and getting the results you want!

Progressive overload targets three of the four aspects of exercise: *intensity*, *time*, and *type*. (The other aspect is frequency—how often you exercise—but you're always going to Shred five times a week.) Each week, you'll bump up one of these three.

- *Intensity:* You'll change up your intensity. Sometimes you will Shred between low and moderate intensity, sometimes between low and high intensity. Pay close attention to the Perceived Exertion Scale that I talk about below: It will show you the way!
- *Time:* All Shredders start out at *just 5* minutes the first week, then increase 5 minutes every week thereafter. At the end of Month 1 you will have worked up to 20 minutes of Shredding. At the end of Month 2, you will be up to 40 minutes of Shredding. By the end of Month 3, you will be up to 60 minutes of Shredding. You will be blown away at how much your body has changed at this point! We top the Shredders off at 60 minutes, because it is important that this program fit into your daily lifestyle. Trust me, at 60 minutes of Shredding you'll be burning so many calories you won't need to increase duration any more!
- *Type:* You'll exercise in different ways. For example, if you've been cycling, you'll switch to basketball. If you're tired of basketball, switch to swimming. If swimming isn't your thing, try dance. Keep

switching up your exercise type as often as you want until you find something you love to do! And then keep switching it up anyway.

INTENSE!

When you exercise, there are a bunch of markers that indicate your fitness level. You sense that your heart rate speeds up. You feel the burn in your muscles. You notice that you breathe faster. That last bit of information is an especially good indicator of your fitness level. You can use it to measure something called *perceived exertion* (PE). This technique is also called the *talk test*, because it judges how much effort it takes for you to exercise based on your ability to talk while working out. The fitter you are, the less effort you exert while doing a particular exercise!

There are all kinds of technology out there that measure your exertion level, from smartphone apps to heart rate monitors, but this basic talk test is one of the fastest and easiest (*and cheapest!*) ways to roughly gauge your exercise intensity any given moment!

PERCIEVED EXERTION LEVEL TALK TEST		
Exertion Score	Exertion Level	Performance
6	light	unbroken conversation, breathing easy
7	moderate	unbroken conversation, breathing heavy
8	brisk	conversation broken, three to four words at a time
9	fast	conversation broken, only single words
10	all-out	cannot talk, panic breathing

Do the talk test and use this PE chart to determine the exercise intensity levels you reach while doing your Shredders. As the duration of your Shredders changes from week to week, so will your intensity. Sometimes you'll Shred between levels 6 and 7, and sometimes you'll Shred between levels 6 and 10!

The beauty of using the PE scale is that you can watch your PE go down as your fitness increases. For example, a light jog might be a level 8

Gimme Five!

Let's be honest. Most of us have a hard time getting motivated to move in the first place, let alone exercise for thirty to sixty minutes every day! Exercise can be intimidating, especially if you are just starting out. Here's the deal: You don't have to exercise for thirty to sixty minutes every day. For many of us, that is an inflated and unattainable promise—and we need to eventually work up to it when we *believe* that we can. That's why the Shredders start out with just five minutes, and increase five minutes every week thereafter. But keep in mind, even when the guidelines call for ten, fifteen, twenty minutes, and beyond, five minutes of Shredding is *always* your promise. It is totally doable, no matter what life throws at you. You can even walk/jog in place for five minutes while watching TV if you have to! If you want to do more, that's awesome and you will just reach your goals faster—but as long as you do just five minutes of Shredding every day, you win.

NOTE: If you have been sedentary for a while and are just starting to move again, feel free to just do five minutes of Shredding every day for two weeks until you are ready to embark upon your 9-Minute Missions.

on your scale now, but in a few weeks, it might fall to level 6. And you might hit level 8 only when you're running. You have to *move faster* to hit your intensity targets . . . but harder work won't feel any different than the lighter work you started with! Before you know it, your friends will have to sprint to keep up with you!

I've engineered the all-new Shredders around the PE principle so they take your fitness to higher and higher levels.

FOUR WAYS TO TEAR IT UP

I've designed four new Shredder protocols, or strategies, that didn't appear in my first book, *Choose to Lose*. These are much more convenient and practical! If this is your first foray into carb cycling, you're one step ahead, starting out with the new and improved Shredders. You can do almost any cardio activity—dancing, spinning, jumping on a trampoline—for your Shredders.

My Shredder plans focus on practicality and simplicity, because the easier they are to follow, the more likely you are to do them! Instead of the three-level (low, medium, and high intensity) Shredders I gave you in *Choose to Lose*, the updated Shredders have only two intensity levels: high and low. What's high intensity and what's low intensity? Easy! Just measure *your personal intensity levels* using the PE chart!

For each protocol—Dirty Two-Thirties, Nasty Nineties, Mighty Minutes, and Thrilling Thirties—I specify the high and low intensities I want you to aim for and the periods of time I want you to exercise at each intensity. You can pick any cardio activity as your Shredder exercise. The workout pattern for all four protocols is the same: Shred at the low-intensity PE level for the period of time shown in the schedule below, then Shred at the high-intensity PE level for the period of time shown in the schedule below. Repeat that circuit until the total duration that I've set for the Shredder has elapsed. That's it!

I've set up a very simple Shredder schedule for you. Each week of the month has its own Shredder, which you'll do five days that week. Here we go!

Pace Yourself Then Push Yourself

As you begin to explore higher levels of intensity, such as Perceived Exertion levels of 8, 9, and 10, it is important to pace yourself early on to make sure you don't fatigue too early. For example, maintaining a PE level of 10 during the Thrilling Thirties for a forty-minute Shredder can wipe out the best athlete in the first fifteen minutes. The key is to push yourself, but pace yourself early on and aim for your max exertion near the end of the Shredder. Use the final five to ten high-intensity intervals to show yourself what you've got!

Shredders - Month at a Glance

WEEK 1	Monday	Tuesday	Wednesday	Thursday	Friday	Saturday	Sunday
Shredders	Dirty Two-Thirties	Dirty Two-Thirties	Dirty Two-Thirties	Dirty Two-Thirties	Dirty Two-Thirties		
Intensity:	2:30 low PE 6 2:30 high PE 7	2:30 low PE 6 2:30 high PE 7	2:30 low PE 6 2:30 high PE 7	2:30 low PE 6 2:30 high PE 7	2:30 low PE 6 2:30 high PE 7	Rest	Rest
Overall Duration:	5 minutes	5 minutes	5 minutes	5 minutes	5 minutes		

WEEK 2	Monday	Tuesday	Wednesday	Thursday	Friday	Saturday	Sunday
Shredders	Nasty Nineties	Nasty Nineties	Nasty Nineties	Nasty Nineties	Nasty Nineties		
Intensity:	90 sec low PE 6 90 sec high PE 8	90 sec low PE 6 90 sec high PE 8	90 sec low PE 6 90 sec high PE 8	90 sec low PE 6 90 sec high PE 8	90 sec low PE 6 90 sec high PE 8	Rest	Rest
Overall Duration:	10 minutes	10 minutes	10 minutes	10 minutes	10 minutes		

WEEK 3	Monday	Tuesday	Wednesday	Thursday	Friday	Saturday	Sunday
Shredders	Mighty Minutes	Mighty Minutes	Mighty Minutes	Mighty Minutes	Mighty Minutes		
Intensity:	1 min low PE 6 1 min high PE 9	1 min low PE 6 1 min high PE 9	1 min low PE 6 1 min high PE 9	1 min low PE 6 1 min high PE 9	1 min low PE 6 1 min high PE 9	Rest	Rest
Overall Duration:	15 minutes	15 minutes	15 minutes	15 minutes	15 minutes		

WEEK 4	Monday	Tuesday	Wednesday	Thursday	Friday	Saturday	Sunday
Shredders	Thrilling Thirties	Thrilling Thirties	Thrilling Thirties	Thrilling Thirties	Thrilling Thirties		
Intensity:	30 sec low PE 6 30 sec high PE 10	30 sec low PE 6 30 sec high PE 10	30 sec low PE 6 30 sec high PE 10	30 sec low PE 6 30 sec high PE 10	30 sec low PE 6 30 sec high PE 10	Rest	Rest
Overall Duration:	20 minutes	20 minutes	20 minutes	20 minutes	20 minutes		

Each week thereafter, add an additional 5 minutes to your overall duration
to work up to about an hour of shredders each day.

VARIETY IS THE SPICE OF SHREDDING

Here's the best part of Shredding. There are so many cardio activities out there that you'll be able to find some you enjoy. Maybe you already have a few favorites! *Any activity* that keeps you moving for a while can be a fat-burning winner. Each and every one can be done at high and low intensity. Pick from exercises you can do at home, at the gym, outdoors, as a sport, or in a group class, and Shred away!

The Dating Game

So many people I meet think they hate exercise, and maybe you're one of them. But *I* know that no one *really* hates exercise—deep down, we're all athletes. Really! You just haven't "met" a form of exercise you love! Trust me: There *is* at least one exercise out there that you can love for the rest of your life. . . . You just don't know it yet! As you begin your journey of transformation, try "dating" every kind of exercise you can imagine doing, from racquetball to hiking, soccer to swimming. Eventually you'll find your perfect match!

At Home

Dodgeball

Jump rope

Playing with your children or dog

Rowing machine

Stationary bike

Tag

Trampoline

Treadmill

At the Gym

Arm ergometer (arm cycle)

Elliptical trainer

Rowing machine

Stair stepper

Stationary or recumbent bike

Treadmill

Outdoors

Bicycling

Bleacher running

Boat rowing

Canoeing

Cross-country skiing

Hiking

Ice skating

Jogging/Running

Kayaking

Nordic walking

Paddle boarding

Power walking (brisk walking)

Rollerblading

Shoveling snow

Snowshoeing

Stair running

Swimming

Walking

Water jogging/running

Sports

Playing sports, it can be difficult to change intensities the way the Shredder protocol suggests, but fortunately changes in intensity are already built in. So play away, knowing that you are getting the most out of your body, and the fat loss results you want!

Basketball

Boxing

Flag football

Hockey

Kickball

Kickboxing

Lacrosse

Martial arts

Racquetball

Soccer

Tennis

Group Classes

Like most sports, group classes move at their own pace—but the high and low intensities happen naturally! Just go with it, and let the instructor guide your Shredding!

Aerobics
Cardio kickboxing
Dancing (hip-hop, salsa, Zumba, etc.)
Spinning
Step aerobics
Water aerobics

FEED YOUR FIRE: THE RECIPES

SUCCESS STORY #6: VANESSA

Food has always been a big part of Vanessa's life, partly, she laughs, because she grew up in an Italian family. The kitchen table was where her family gathered to talk and enjoy one another—and there was *always* something to eat.

But there was another reason Vanessa ate: When she was six years old she was diagnosed with a learning disorder and a speech impediment. The kids at school teased her and called her names, and she often went home in tears. Vanessa turned to food for comfort. Food made her feel safe inside, it didn't judge her, and it was always there for her.

By the time she was twelve, Vanessa weighed over two hundred pounds. By the time she started high school she weighed three-hundred–plus. Her parents tried to help her lose weight; they even enrolled her in Weight Watchers. At the same time, her mother would tell her that she was beautiful, and that should never let anyone tell her she wasn't. But Vanessa sure didn't *feel* beautiful.

Vanessa tried every diet out there, but her weight kept going up and up. Even though she was popular, she felt like a horrible person trapped in a disgusting body. She couldn't fit onto amusement park rides, and she once broke an auditorium seat, making all the kids laugh. She felt helpless and insecure. When her family moved to Las Vegas, she hoped to leave all that behind.

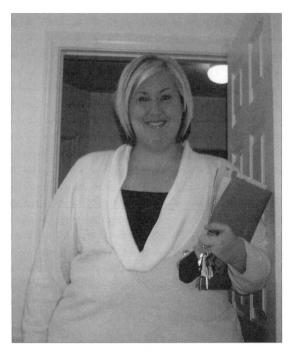

In high school, Vanessa started having severe panic attacks, and kept eating her way through her problems. Finally, miserable and traumatized, she dropped out of school. She didn't go to her prom or earn a cap and gown. Instead, she got her GED and started college—even though she couldn't fit into a desk! She felt trapped in her own body.

Then something happened. When Vanessa was twenty, she got a job at a tanning salon, and within three months she became its number one salesperson! The other employees were beautiful and fit, but the clients loved *her*. Vanessa began to respect herself and see her own charm. She began to believe what her mother told her about being beautiful, and for six more years she rocked the tanning salon.

But when she was twenty-six, her mother died unexpectedly. Devastated, Vanessa lost her grip on her newfound self-esteem. For the next few years she struggled with her weight, her work, her love life—everything. She hit 376 pounds. Yet she was determined to turn her life around. She earned her nursing assistant degree and started working in an acute care hospital.

Some of her patients were morbidly obese, which shook Vanessa deeply. She knew that if she didn't change, she'd end up just like them. A light flickered to life in her mind. She'd been watching *Extreme Makeover: Weight Loss Edition* and decided to try out for a spot on the show. She wasn't selected, but Vanessa realized *she* had to do the hard work of putting her life back together—no one else was going to do it for her. So she started the transformation of a lifetime!

Vanessa threw herself into my program of diet and exercise. Working out hurt at first, and it was tough to be the heaviest person at her gym. Eating right was a challenge, especially since meals had often been a social event for her. Dinner and drinks had to be a no-no for the first few months! Never comfortable in the kitchen, Vanessa had to *learn* how to put her meals together—in advance. She took her food to the hospital, but when she was working thirteen-hour days, she found it difficult to eat five times a day, every three hours.

But it was a lot harder to tackle her deeper food issues and break her self-destructive emotional habits. Vanessa knew she had to change her mind-set about food and accept that she could feel happy and secure without eating all the time. As she kept at it, she began to transform into a new person. Instead of the off-the-wall, plus-size personality she'd been trying so hard to keep up, she started to become . . . Vanessa. She felt that her life had just begun!

Before long, Vanessa realized that she felt great when she ate chicken breasts and veggies instead of pasta and cupcakes. Now she drinks protein shakes instead of alcohol. Instead of eating a breakfast of bagels and cream cheese standing at the nurses' station, she eats yogurt

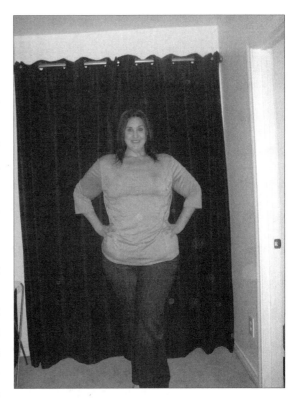

and fresh fruit sitting at her kitchen table, fifteen minutes after she wakes up. Vanessa *craves* healthy food and really enjoys her five meals a day. She knows that if she makes a bad food choice she can still finish the day right. A bad food day doesn't have to turn into a bad food week!

And Vanessa loves to work out. She's still the largest person in her spin class, but now she spins in the front row instead of the back! Every day she pushes herself, and she keeps her workouts fun by switching up her routine. In 2013 she plans to run her first half marathon and earn her personal trainer and life coach certifications.

It took Vanessa six months to lose her first 115 pounds and bring her weight down to 261. She's still working, and nothing's going to stop her from reaching her goal weight. She feels truly alive and full of energy—body and soul. Happier and stronger than ever, she never looks back, only ahead. Now she's looking forward to helping people just like her realize they can do *anything* they set their mind to. Her motto is "If I can do it, anyone can!"

Feeding Your Fire

Heidi and I love the old phrase, "Give a man a fish, feed him for a day; teach a man to fish, feed him for a lifetime." That's just what we're going to do for you in this chapter. Super-easy and super-smart, our recipes are truly *empowering*, both in your kitchen and in your entire life transformation. Even better, after you read this chapter, you're not only going to have a whole bunch of great new carb-cycling recipes, you're going to have high-level food intelligence that will help you maintain and enhance your transformation—for a lifetime!

Cooking! Sound like more than you can handle? Nuh-uh. To be honest, Heidi and I aren't into cooking big, elaborate meals. Like most folks, we just don't have enough time. We're always on the go, whether it is running the kids to their daily activities or taking a crowd of people through a workout in the middle of Times Square! But we know that to maintain our healthy lifestyle we need to prepare and eat our own food. We spent the last few years perfecting the fastest and easiest ways to prepare the foods we need, and I'm going to share our secrets with you.

We *love* convenience. When it comes to food preparation, we want it *fast, easy, and fun!* Our recipes are definitely not complicated, confusing, or time-consuming. They use familiar ingredients that you can find in your local supermarket, and we definitely don't expect you to know any fancy culinary techniques or own any expensive kitchen equipment. If you're not big on cooking, or you just don't have much time to spare, rest assured that our recipes will get you in and out of your kitchen in a flash.

Whether you're a novice in the kitchen or a pro, you're about to learn how to use food to take control of your body and your weight loss. We'll show you how to put together a dish or a meal using healthy ingredients, figure out your right portion sizes, and, just as important, add zest to your food with delicious techniques. This simple info is all you're going to need to whip up effective, enjoyable meals that help you achieve your goals!

We do recipes a little bit differently around here, so you won't just get a list of ingredients, a set of directions, and a "good luck." This chapter's packed with tips and how-to's on food storage, portioning, advance preparation, bulk preparation, food substitutions, and the like. We lay out our food categories—proteins, carbohydrates, veggies, and fats—in easy-to-read charts, so you'll quickly get the big picture on nutrition. And we follow a simple model for all the recipes: Each is based on a protein foundation and includes a high- and low-carb variation.

If you want to take carb-cycle cooking up to the next level (but you don't have to!), you're going to love this! That's because you're getting the building blocks of *meal creation*, a process that goes beyond making a tasty breakfast burrito. I'm going to clue you in on how to tailor your meals to *your own tastes* and requirements. Once you learn the tricks of combining ingredients, adapting recipes, and cooking quick meals that keep your mouth and your metabolism happy, you'll be on your way to success!

All of our recipes are wonderfully *customizable and interchangeable*, so you've got endless possibilities for designing your very own carb-cycling dishes and menus. The recipes note the category of each ingredient, so you'll be able to analyze your favorite recipes and adapt them while making sure your tweaks follow the carb-cycling rules. Choose a different protein for a recipe, change a side to turn your high-carb meal into a low-carb meal, invent your own dishes with smart foods and techniques—before you know it, you'll be a virtuoso at mixing and matching ingredients for maximum flavor and benefit any day of the week!

"Yikes!" you say? "All I want are easy recipes for good, healthy food that'll help me lose weight!" Don't worry. I guarantee you'll get carb cycling right just by following our simple food prep instructions, step by step. But eating won't be boring! Even if you stick with the most basic of the basics, you're going to enjoy these meals!

You *Can* Afford to Eat Healthy

I can hear it now: "But Chris, all this healthy food's going to be expensive!" You ready for my comeback? Some of the *cheapest* foods per serving are the fruits, eggs, grains, and veggies that I want you to eat! In fact, Heidi and I each eat for $6 to $12 a day . . . really! Eating processed, fast, and junk food has actually been costing you more than the real, whole food you'll be eating on your carb cycle. Not to mention the long-term impact on your health. Think of the doctor's bills you won't have to pay.

So many healthy foods have really reasonable prices, but you can *save even more* by clipping coupons and keeping an eye out for sales at your supermarket. Don't forget store brands, either. A lot of the food that's sold under supermarket labels comes from the exact same producers as the brand-name stuff does!

Sure, some healthy foods can be expensive, especially protein. Don't panic if one of our recipes calls for a meat or fish that isn't in your budget. You can always use a less expensive, nutritionally comparable variety. For example, some cuts of steak can be pretty pricey, but you can *save about a third off*, more or less, by choosing less swanky cuts (e.g., eye round, flatiron, or some types of sirloin). And it just so happens that some of the less expensive cuts are a lot tastier and a lot leaner! It's the same story with fish: Pound for pound, large shrimp cost more than small shrimp, salmon's cheaper than tuna, etc. Make budget-friendly protein choices; buy a little extra of whatever's on sale and freeze it to use later.

There's been a greenmarket boom in the United States over the past ten years or so, but maybe you've always figured shopping at one of them would be costly. Believe it or not, most veggies and fruits sold at farmers' markets are less expensive than they are in the supermarket! And if you're into organic food, greenmarket prices are *a lot* lower. Plus, the food you get from the local farms that sell this way is much fresher—therefore, richer in nutrients—than supermarket produce. There's bound to be a weekly farmers' market near you.

Some herbs and spices are very expensive, mostly because of packaging. You can save significantly at Mexican, Asian, and other international grocery stores, or in the ethnic section at your supermarket, where herbs and spices often come in plain cellophane bags. Many large supermarket chains now sell herbs and spices under the supermarket's own label, without the brand-name extras (which you don't need). Another great source for these flavorings can be your local health food store, which might carry herbs and spices in bulk, with no packaging at all.

These stores also sell healthy grains, like brown rice and rolled oats, plus many varieties of granola, in bulk. Whether for grains or spices, there are two big advantages to shopping at health food stores: First, many of their products are minimally processed and grown without pesticides; and second, you can buy exactly as much as you want instead of the amount preloaded into commercial packaging.

How Much Can I Eat?

For weight loss, not only is it essential to eat the right foods, it's essential that you eat the *right amount* of food. It boils down to calories. Uggh. Calculating calories is no fun, and it's easy to get it wrong, but you need to watch 'em: They measure how much fuel you're putting into your body. Even a little bit of extra fuel can quickly accumulate in your body, so it's important to make sure portions are right *for you.*

There are all sorts of new smartphone apps that count calories, and some of them are amazing! But here's the catch. You have to *use* them for them to work. Let's get real: Most of us need something simpler. You could buy a calorie-counting app for your phone, but there's a much more convenient way—a low-tech way—to guesstimate portions: Use your hands! That's right. Hand portioning is smart, easy to remember and easy to use wherever you go.

- *Proteins:* Your portion is the size and thickness of the palm of your hand.
- *Carbs:* Your portion is the size of your clenched fist.
- *Veggies:* Your portion is the size of two of your clenched fists, but you can eat as many veggies as you like!
- *Fats:* Your portion is the size of your thumb, from the base up.
- *Sauces, dressings, and condiments:* Your portion should be no larger than the size of your index and middle finger, from the base up.

Many diets ask you to weigh all of your food. If you can actually make it part of your lifestyle, more power to you—you'll get great results! But who's got the time or patience to put it all on a scale? Good news: Hand portioning makes weight loss and maintenance *way easier* today and for the rest of your life. This explains why most of our recipes don't measure quantities in terms of ounces or pounds.

But FYI, here's how hand portioning equates to cooking measurements:

CARB-CYCLING PORTION CONVERSION: AVERAGE PER-MEAL ESTIMATES				
	Protein	Carbs	Veggies	Fats
Hand portion	1 Palm	1 Fist	2 Fists	1 Thumb
Men's Portion	5 Oz	1.5 Cups	3 Cups	2 Tbsp
Women's Portion	3 Oz	1 Cup	2 Cups	1 Tbsp

Take Your Calories in Hand

Although hand portioning is fast and easy, it's not absolutely precise. Each time you measure a thumb-size portion of peanut butter, it's going to be slightly different from the portion you measured last time. Plus, the portion conversion chart above is based on the *average* hand sizes of men and women, which are probably different from the size of your hands. Some women have bigger hands than others, and the same goes for men! So you might need to adjust your hand portions.

But even if your hand size yielded the exact portions shown in the conversion chart above, portions of various foods have *different calorie counts*. That is, different ingredients within the same food category (proteins, carbs, veggies, or fats) are more or less calorie-dense than others. For instance, a palm-size, five-ounce portion of ground beef has more calories than the same amount of chicken breast. So you need a way to translate your paws into calories.

Using your hands to measure your portions puts you in the ballpark, because people who have bigger hands—in general, that's men—end up with bigger portions. Perfect! Men need to eat more calories than women. How much more? Well, women should cycle between 1,200 and 1,500 calories daily, while men should cycle between 1,500 and 2,000 calories.

Beware! Somewhere along your weight-loss journey, you'll be tempted to speed the process by *eating fewer calories* than I recommend. Bad idea. If you take in too few calories, your body will get the signal to protect its fuel reserves. Your metabolism will *slow down*, and your weight-loss mission will be derailed—or even stopped. To prevent this from happening, get your calories!

Bottom line, you've got to make sure you're getting close to the *right number of calories every day*. As long as you're in the ballpark, you're going to get results. To determine the approximate number of calories you're consuming daily, go to the next section and check out the list of recommended carb-cycling foods, which we've measured out into 100-calorie portions. The size of a 100-calorie portion of any of the approved foods gives you an idea for how your hand portion sizes up.

At the start of your carb-cycling program, take a little time to see how your hand portions translate into numerical measurements. It's actually kind of fun. Put together a palm-size portion of a protein, a fist-size portion of a carb, a double-fist portion of veggies, and a thumb's worth of fat. Put

Tuning Up Your Taste Buds

If you're like a lot of my clients, you aren't used to eating healthy food. And like them, when you first make the switch to real, whole, fresh food, you might think it's kind of bland. Here's why: The intense sweeteners, chemicals, and additives you've been eating have actually *weakened your taste buds*. You can hardly taste real food anymore! The more damage that has been done, the sweeter and saltier food has to be to taste good to you, so you eat more and more heavily seasoned food. Your taste buds are attacked again and again.

But there's good news: *You can repair the damage.* Tough it out for one week of healthy eating, and your taste buds will heal and grow back! The good stuff will taste good, and the bad stuff will taste . . . bad. Go ahead and try some of your old favorites, and I guarantee they'll taste sweeter, saltier, and fattier. Before long, artificially flavored food will be way too salty and sweet, and fatty food will taste pretty darn greasy!

those portions into measuring cups or spoons, and see how much of each food you end up with. Then do it backward: Measure out the recommended portion of each food and see how it compares to your hand size. Cool, huh? This will help you portion more accurately with your hands. Remember, once you've got your hand measurements dialed in, you'll have them for life!

Another way to get a grip on portioning is, for a week or so at the beginning of your carb-cycling program, to use measuring spoons and cups to dish out your ingredients. It might be a pain, but it only takes a few extra seconds, and soon you'll get the hang of portioning with your hands instead of utensils. From then on you'll have a portable tool for measuring out the right number of calories each day, and you'll be on your way to your weight-loss goal!

What Can I Eat?

Ah, finally, the nitty-gritty info you've been waiting for: The List. Here's where you find out what you're going to be able to eat on the carb-cycling plan. We call them *smart foods*—smart proteins, smart carbs, smart veggies, and smart fats. We even list smart condiments and smart beverages! And we show you how much of each item is in a 100-calorie portion. Stick with smart foods and portions, and you're good to go!

Recommended Carb-Cycling Smart Foods and 100-Calorie Portions

Protein	Approximately 100 Calories
Beef	
Cube Steak	2.5 oz
Flank Steak (lean)	2 oz
Roast Beef (low-sodium)	3 oz
Round Steak	2.5 oz
Sirloin Steak (extra lean)	2 oz
Venison/Elk	2 oz

Protein	Approximately 100 Calories
Dairy	
Cottage Cheese	½ cup
Egg Substitutes	1 cup
Egg Whites	4 Whites
Greek Yogurt (nonfat, plain)	¾ cup
Lean Ground Meats	
Ground Beef (extra lean)	2 oz
Ground Chicken Breast (raw)	4 oz
Ground Turkey (99% fat-free, raw)	3 oz
Poultry	
Chicken (canned—high sodium warning!)	4 oz
Duck Breast	2 oz
Foster Farms Chicken Breast (skinless)	3.5 oz
Foster Farms Chicken Thighs (skinless)	3 oz
Turkey Breast (low-sodium deli)	3 oz
Turkey Breast (skinless, *not deli*)	2.5 oz
Powdered	
Whey, Egg, Soy, Rice, Hemp	1 scoop
Fish	
Salmon (canned)	3.5 oz
Salmon (fillet)	2 oz
Sardines	4 sardines (52g)
Tuna (canned)	3 oz
Tuna (fillet)	3 oz
White Fish (branzino, catfish, cod, flounder, grouper, haddock, halibut, pollock, sea bass, snapper, sole, swordfish, trout, tilapia, tilefish)	2.5 oz

Protein	Approximately 100 Calories
Shellfish	
Clams (raw)	5 oz
Lobster/Shrimp	4 oz
Vegetable Protein	
Tempeh	2 oz
Texturized Vegetable Protein	2 oz
Tofu	4 oz
White Meat	
Pork Tenderloin	2.5

Carbs	Approximately 100 Calories
Breads	
Brown Rice tortillas	1 tortilla
Corn Tortillas	1½ tortillas
Ezekiel 4.9 Breads	1 slice
Ezekiel 4.9 English Muffin	½ muffin
Ezekiel 4.9 Tortillas	¾ tortilla
Whole-Grain Bread	1 slice
Cereal	
All-Bran	½ cup
Fiber One	¾ cup
Kashi Go Lean	½ cup
Kashi Good Friends Cereal	½ cup
Kashi Heart to Heart	¾ cup
Low-Fat Granola	½ cup
Old-Fashioned Oatmeal (cooked)	¾ cup
Steel-Cut Oatmeal (cooked)	¾ cup

Carbs	Approximately 100 Calories
Grains	
Amaranth	½ cup
Barley	½ cup
Bran	½ cup
Buckwheat	½ cup
Brown Rice (cooked)	½ cup
Millet (uncooked)	⅛ cup
Oats (steel-cut and cooked)	⅔ cup
Popcorn (air-popped, no oil)	3 cups
Quinoa	½ cup
Wild Rice	½ cup
Legumes	
Beans (boiled or low-sodium canned)	½ cup
Lentils (cooked and boiled)	½ cup
Soybeans (edamame)	¼ cup
Soy Nuts (roasted, lightly salted)	3 Tbsp
Pasta	
Brown Rice Pasta	½ cup
Couscous	½ cup
Whole grain pasta	½ cup
Root Vegetables	
Beets	1½ cups
Carrots	2 cups
Parsnips	1 cup
Potatoes (russet/red/gold)	¾ cup
Rutabagas	2 cups
Sweet Potatoes/Yams	⅔ cup
Starchy Veggies	
Corn (fresh)	⅔ cup
Peas (fresh)	1 cup

Fruit	Approximately 100 Calories
Fresh	
Apples	1½ apples
Apricots	6 apricots
Banana	1
Berries (e.g., blackberries, blueberries, cherries, raspberries, strawberries)	1½ cups
Grapes	1½ cups
Grapefruit	1 grapefruit
Kiwifruit	4 kiwifruits
Lemons	5 lemons
Limes	5 limes
Oranges/Tangerines	1 orange/tangerine
Mangoes	1 cup
Melons	1½ cups
Papayas	2 cups
Peaches/Nectarines	2 large peaches
Pears	1 pear
Pineapple	1⅓ cup
Plums	3½ plums

Veggies	Approximately 100 Calories
Artichokes	2 medium
Asparagus	3½ cups
Bok Choy	1 head
Broccoli	4 cups
Broccoli Rabe	4 cups
Brussels Sprouts	2½ cups
Cabbage	4 cups
Cauliflower	4 cups
Celery	5 cups
Chard	10 leaves
Collard Greens	10 cups
Cucumber	4 medium
Endive	1 head

Veggies	Approximately 100 Calories
Eggplant	5 cups
Fennel	4 cups
Garlic	20 cloves
Green Beans/Wax Beans	75 beans
Kale	3 cups
Leeks	2 leeks
Mushrooms	20 large
Mustard Greens	7 cups
Okra	3 cups
Onions	2 medium
Peppers	4 medium
Parsley	4 cups
Radicchio	10 cups
Radishes	5 cups
Rhubarb	10 stalks
Salad Greens (e.g., arugula, romaine, other lettuces)	12 cups
Scallions/Green Onions	10 cups
Shallots	10 Tbsp
Snow Peas	70 pods
Spinach	10 cups
Sprouts	1½ cups
Squash	3 medium
Tomatoes (fresh)	6½ medium
Turnips	3 medium
Zucchini	2 large

Fats	70–100 Calories
Dairy	
Blue Cheese	1 oz
Brie	1 oz
Cream Cheese	2 Tbsp
Egg Yolk	2
Feta Cheese	1 oz

Fats	70–100 Calories
Goat Cheese	1 oz
Heavy Whipping Cream	2 Tbsp
Mozzarella	1 oz
Parmesan	1 oz
Romano	1 oz
Sliced Cheeses (e.g., Cheddar, Colby, Gouda, Havarti, Monterey Jack, Muenster, Swiss)	1 oz (1 oz = 1 slice)
Sliced Cheeses (low-fat)	2 oz (1 oz = 1 slice)

Dressings

Creamy Dressing (low-fat)	2 Tbsp
Creamy Dressing (regular)	1 Tbsp
Mayonnaise (regular)	2 Tbsp

Fruit

Avocado	$\frac{1}{3}$ cup
Olives (large, brine-cured)	13

Nuts and Seeds

Almond Butter (with salt)	1 Tbsp
Almonds (raw, chopped)	1½ Tbsp
Peanut Butter (with salt)	1 Tbsp
Pecans (raw, chopped)	1½ Tbsp
Sesame Butter (tahini)	1¼ Tbsp
Sesame Seeds	2 Tbsp
Sunflower Seeds	1½ Tbsp
Walnuts (raw, chopped)	1½ Tbsp

Oils

Flaxseed Oil	1 Tbsp
Olive Oil	1 Tbsp

Flavorings	30–50 Calories
Butter Spray	5 sprays
Balsamic Vinaigrette	2 Tbsp
Chili Paste	2 Tbsp
Chili Sauce	2 Tbsp
Extracts (e.g., almond, peppermint, vanilla)	unlimited
Fat-Free Balsamic Vinaigrette	2 Tbsp
Fat-Free French Dressing	2 Tbsp
Fat-Free Mayo/Low-Fat Mayo	2 Tbsp
Hummus	2 Tbsp
Hot Sauce (e.g., Tabasco)	3 tsp
Ketchup (low-sodium)	2 Tbsp
Lemon Juice	3 oz
Lime Juice	3 oz
Low-Fat Italian Dressing (Newman's Own LITE)	2 Tbsp
Low-Sodium Chicken Broth	1 cup
Low-Sodium Soy Sauce	2 tsp
Marinara Sauce (Newman's Own)	½ cup
Mustard	3 tsp
Salsa (Newman's Own All-Natural)	½ cup
Stevia, Xylitol, Erythritol	unlimited
Tomato Paste	3 Tbsp
Tomato Sauce	½ cup
Vinegar (e.g., cider, red, or white-wine)	unlimited
Worcestershire Sauce (high sodium warning!)	2 tbsp

Beverages	100 Calories
Almond milk (unsweetened)	2½ cups
Coconut Water (pure)	2 cups
Coffee (black)	unlimited
Soy milk (unsweetened)	1¼ cup
Tea (black)	unlimited

Beverages	100 Calories
Tea (green)	unlimited
Tea (herbal)	unlimited
Tomato juice	2½ cups
Water (flat or sparkling)	unlimited

Bulk-Prep Your Food

Let's be honest: Unless you love to cook, you've got a slew of better ways to spend your time than sweating in the kitchen before each meal. A terrific way to make carb cycling easier is to shop for and prepare and cook large quantities of ingredients *before you'll need them* to assemble your

Steer Clear of Sodium!

Most processed food contains incredibly huge quantities of sodium. The evil eats come in all forms—commercially packaged stuff might be frozen, refrigerated, bottled, canned, bagged, or boxed; deli meats and "fresh" prepared foods are big offenders. While sodium itself is a necessary electrolyte and an absolute requirement for your health, you've got to consume it in moderation. Sodium enhances flavor and preserves food, but manufacturers add such massive quantities to most processed foods that your health takes a beating if you eat them. In the long term, frequent intake of high-sodium food can lead to hypertension, damaging your arteries. In the short term, too much sodium in your system can cause substantial *water retention and bloating*. These short-term effects mess with your weekly weigh-ins, when you'll see false weight gains on your scale! What to do? When you shop, stick with genuinely clean and fresh foods, and when you *have* to buy processed stuff, try to find low-sodium options. Keep away from processed food whenever possible!

meals. It won't just free up your time: Keeping cooked, pre-portioned, pre-marinated meats and veggies, and pre-mixed dressings and sauces in your fridge and freezer lets you gather the ingredients for any recipe at a moment's notice. Fewer trips to the supermarket and simpler, quicker meal prep will help you eat right and stay on track with your carb-cycling program. Plan ahead so your food's ready when you are!

Each of our recipes includes ingredient measurements for making different numbers of servings. The numbers 1, 2, 4, 6, or 8 at the top of each recipe tell you how many portions you'll get using the ingredient quantities listed below each number. Visiting the supermarket just once to buy what you need for several meals reduces the stress and time that goes into shopping. And prepping these larger quantities of ingredients in a single session—more food than you'll be using right away—will *save you a ton of time* later on. The multiplied measurements also allow you to adapt the recipes to serve everyone at a family or group meal, or to take the dish to a potluck! After all, carb-cycling food isn't diet food: It's everyday food made in healthy ways. If you don't tell them, your family might not even know they're eating healthy!

Now, you aren't restricted to eating only the dishes we give you here. You can use the recipes in my first book, *Choose to Lose*, or those that you find in other sources or make up yourself—as long as they *use only smart foods, in the right portions*. If you want to prepare those in bulk, you'll probably have to figure out how much of each ingredient you need to use if you multiply the recipes to serve more people. With all of those ¾ teaspoons and ⅓ cups, it's a pain to do the math! So we've created a handy chart that gives you all the multiplied measurements you're likely to need. Turn to Appendix D: "Multiple-Serving Measurement Chart" in the back of the book.

We like to get ready for about four days of meals at a time by having a cooking marathon. Heidi and I usually bulk-prep our food on Sundays and Wednesdays; sometimes that changes depending on our work schedules. So here's what you do: Start by choosing two or three similar recipes and then find the *ingredients they have in common*—say, if they both call for chicken breast. For those shared ingredients, take a look at the quantities you need to make the number of servings you want. Add up the numbers, make a shopping list that includes the amount you need for each ingredient, and head out to the store. Back at home, lay the ingredients out on the counter, then slice and peel and chop for all the recipes at the same time.

Once you've prepped all the ingredients for one of your recipes, get it started on the stove or in the oven. While that's cooking, finish prepping the ingredients for your second recipe. If you can handle cooking two dishes at once, get recipe number two started, then go through the same routine for recipe number three—or slow it down and wait awhile. Keep an eye on everything at once! You don't want to end up with burned food.

When you're done cooking, *allow your food to cool* unless you'll be eating it right away. Portion it out and put it into plastic Baggies or storage containers. Label your containers using tape or a permanent marker so you can quickly pick out what you want when you're ready to eat it. Depending on when you plan to eat your pre-prepped food, store it in the fridge or freezer. I usually use some of my portions for that day's meals and store the rest in the fridge or freezer.

You may never have heard about bulk-prepping before, but fitness professionals and athletes have been doing it for decades. If you want to eat every three hours, you have to have the right foods available at the right

It's All Cool!

Don't be afraid to buy frozen meat, poultry, or fish! It's perfectly tasty and easy to handle, and comes in very handy when you're making your meals. Many frozen meats are already portioned just right, but before you get cooking, *always check that the portion is the size of your palm*. If it's too big, cut it down.

Also, you don't have to defrost if you want to marinate! Put a portion in a plastic bag along with the marinade ingredients, seal it, and give it a shake, then reopen the bag to *squeeze out as much air as you can* before resealing it and popping it back in the freezer. Or you can put the bag in the fridge to defrost and marinate the meat overnight.

times. Cooking a meal from scratch every three hours is simply unreasonable. But if you make your food in advance, in bulk, the food you need will be there for you exactly when you need it! For Heidi and me, bulk food prep usually takes thirty to seventy-five minutes per session, but it saves *hours* over the next several days. Such a small time investment up front can ensure nutrition success over the next four days. It is a win, every time.

The Possibilities Are Endless

All of my recipes, based on a foundation of protein, offer high- and low-carb-day versions. But there are loads of other ways to add variety to your meals. There's no reason to hold back: It's okay to incorporate more than one type of protein, carb, or fat into a single meal! If you want to, you can mix two proteins together in a recipe—say, turkey and tofu—instead of using just one. The same goes for carbs and fats. The key is that you *don't exceed your portion sizes*. You could, for instance, use a wild rice–lentils combo that adds up to your fist-size carb portion. Go ahead and experiment. New ingredient combos mean new recipe flavors, so you'll never get bored.

Another way to engineer your meals to suit your personal tastes is to be creative when following the instructions "serve with your favorite carb/vegetable side dish" that you'll find in most entrée recipes. Go to town—serve *a different side dish* every time! Just make sure your carb portions don't exceed your fist size.

And you can keep mixing it up by using different herbs, spices, oils, sauces, and condiments. Each recipe includes one or more ingredients in the flavoring category, but you can always use another flavor. In fact, herbs, spices, and other kinds of flavoring are your greatest cooking assets: You can *give almost any dish a different spin* simply by switching up your flavorings. The options are unlimited when it comes to herbs, spices, and calorie-free condiments, but you've got to watch your portions of other condiments, as well as oils and sauces, because they do have calories. No worries about zing, though. Even a little bit of seasoning can deliver a whole lot of flavor!

As you experiment with ingredient combinations, mix-and-match side dishes and all the exciting flavorings out there, you'll quickly *discover your tastes*. Once you know which way your taste buds swing, feel free to substitute ingredients to your heart's content and whip up side dishes that suit your food moods. Increase your flavorings if you prefer more robust food, or decrease them if you like things milder. A little more or less of any single ingredient won't ruin most of the recipes, so go with experimentation and creativity and keep things exciting!

No Meat? No Problem!

Don't worry if you're a vegan or vegetarian! The beauty of the *Choose More, Lose More* recipes is that tofu can be substituted into any meal! Plain tofu is relatively flavorless, so it can be seasoned any way you want to add a whole new kick to your meals.

Tofu is basically coagulated and pressed soy milk, and it packs a heck of a protein punch. It comes in two main forms: Firm and silken. Firm tofu is great for a stir fry and mixing into meals, and silken tofu is fantastic for tofu steaks.

If you are new to preparing tofu, here's a quick and easy guide:

1. Most tofu is packed in water, so your first step is to get the water out. Cut the tofu into portion-sized blocks or strips and place it between two paper towels.
2. Set the tofu on a plate and put another plate on top of it. Use a soup can or some other weight on top of the plate to add pressure to the tofu. Let it rest there for 15–30 minutes, or simply add some pressure yourself for a minute or two. This squeezes the water out.
3. Cook it up! Tofu is extremely versatile. It will soak up any flavor you marinate or season it with. You can grill it, lightly sauté it, bake it, or even toast it if you like. Get creative and enjoy your tofu!

THE RECIPES

PROTEIN SHAKE

	Ingredients	1 Portion	2 Portions
Protein*	protein powder (whey, pea, rice, soy, or egg)	1 scoop	2 scoops
Flavoring	SweetLeaf flavored stevia drops (berry, grape, orange, vanilla, banana, cinnamon etc.)	1–5 drops	1–5 drops
	unsweetened vanilla almond milk OR cold water	1 cup	2 cups

*Every portion of protein in these recipes is appropriate for women. They are near (not exactly) 100 calories per portion of protein. Men will increase slightly based on their daily caloric needs that are laid out in earlier chapters. A good rule of thumb: Men should eat around 1.5 times the portion of women.

Combine protein powder with unsweetened almond milk or cold water. Shake well in shaker bottle or mix with 1 cup ice in blender until smooth. Flavor with stevia drops if desired. Enjoy!

MAKE THIS A LOW CARB MEAL

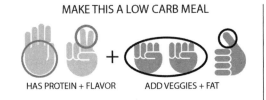

HAS PROTEIN + FLAVOR   ADD VEGGIES + FAT

MAKE THIS A HIGH CARB MEAL

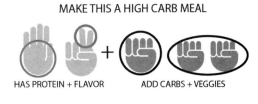

HAS PROTEIN + FLAVOR   ADD CARBS + VEGGIES

Fats	Enjoy with a portion of nuts, such as pecans, almonds, or walnuts, OR blend in a portion of peanut butter.	Carb	Enjoy with a portion of your favorite fruit, whole grain toast, or oatmeal.

Veggies	In vanilla shakes, blend in 3 cups of spinach and kale combined and 1 carrot.	Veggies	In vanilla shakes, blend in 3 cups of spinach and kale combined and 1 carrot.

THE BASIC OMELET

	Ingredients	1 Portion	2 Portions
Protein	Egg whites	4 whites	8 whites
Veggie	Chopped bell peppers, onions, tomato, spinach, mushrooms—whatever you like!	1 cup	2 cups
Prep	Olive oil in spritzer bottle*	1 spritz	2 spritzes

*While I have found that a spritzer bottle is a convenient way to add oils to meals, it's not necessary for these recipes. If you don't have one, don't worry! Just add a few drops everywhere I say "spritz"—or use an olive oil cooking spray.

A great way to start your day off is with an egg-white omelet. Eggs are one of the least expensive sources of protein. They make for a great high-carb breakfast when combined with fruit, oatmeal, whole grain toast, or tortillas. Plus, omelets are also great for dinner! Once or twice a week, bring some variety to your meals with an omelet. Just make sure to watch your ingredients to ensure a proper ratio of proteins/carbs/veggies or proteins/fats/veggies, depending on whether it's a high-carb day or a low-carb day.

Do-Ahead Tip: Put the egg whites in a sandwich-size zip-top bag and add your favorite omelet ingredients. Seal the bag and gently massage it to mix ingredients together. Use within twenty-four hours; simply pour the mixture into a heated pan with a spritz of the olive oil.

1. Separate egg whites from yolks. In a small bowl, whisk egg whites for about 45 seconds.
2. Heat oil in a medium nonstick pan over medium-high heat. Add the egg-white mixture to the pan. Slowly turn the pan to ensure the egg mixture covers the entire bottom.
3. Using a rubber spatula, gently lift the edges of the omelet, tilting the pan so the remaining liquid can go beneath the egg and begin to cook.
4. Let the omelet finish cooking (when egg whites have set) on one side, then using a spatula carefully flip it over to continue cooking on other side.
5. If you are adding ingredients, sprinkle them onto the center of the omelet and continue cooking. Fold the omelet in half to enclose the added ingredients. Enjoy!

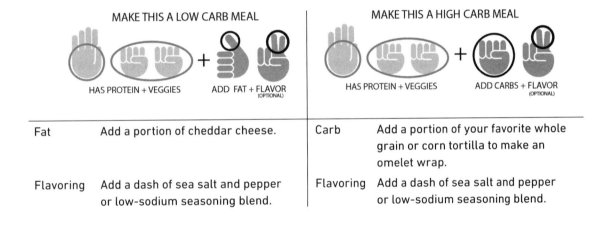

	MAKE THIS A LOW CARB MEAL		MAKE THIS A HIGH CARB MEAL	
Fat	Add a portion of cheddar cheese.	Carb	Add a portion of your favorite whole grain or corn tortilla to make an omelet wrap.	
Flavoring	Add a dash of sea salt and pepper or low-sodium seasoning blend.	Flavoring	Add a dash of sea salt and pepper or low-sodium seasoning blend.	

CLASSIC HAM OMELET

	Ingredients	1 Portion	2 Portions
Protein	Egg whites	3 whites	6 whites
	Ham, low-sodium, chopped	2 Tbsp	4 Tbsp
Veggie	Mushrooms, sliced	½ cup	1 cup
	Tomato, chopped	2 Tbsp	4 Tbsp

Follow directions for The Basic Omelet above.

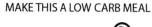
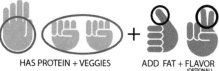

MAKE THIS A LOW CARB MEAL

HAS PROTEIN + VEGGIES   ADD FAT + FLAVOR (OPTIONAL)

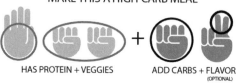

MAKE THIS A HIGH CARB MEAL

HAS PROTEIN + VEGGIES   ADD CARBS + FLAVOR (OPTIONAL)

Fat	Add a portion of cheddar cheese.	
Flavoring	Add a dash of sea salt and pepper or low-sodium seasoning blend.	

Carb	Add a portion of your favorite fruit.
Flavoring	Add a dash of sea salt and pepper or low-sodium seasoning blend.

SPANISH OMELET

	Ingredients	1 Portion	2 Portions
Protein	Egg whites	4 whites	8 whites
Veggie	Onion, chopped	2 Tbsp	4 Tbsp
	Red and/or green bell pepper, chopped	2 Tbsp	4 Tbsp

Follow directions for The Basic Omelet above.

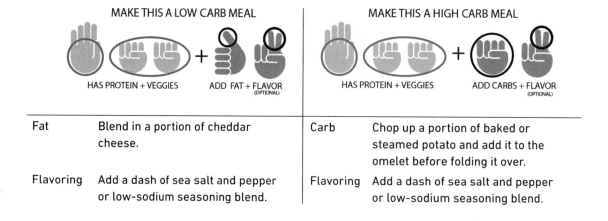

MAKE THIS A LOW CARB MEAL

HAS PROTEIN + VEGGIES   ADD FAT + FLAVOR (OPTIONAL)

MAKE THIS A HIGH CARB MEAL

HAS PROTEIN + VEGGIES   ADD CARBS + FLAVOR (OPTIONAL)

Fat	Blend in a portion of cheddar cheese.
Flavoring	Add a dash of sea salt and pepper or low-sodium seasoning blend.

Carb	Chop up a portion of baked or steamed potato and add it to the omelet before folding it over.
Flavoring	Add a dash of sea salt and pepper or low-sodium seasoning blend.

DENVER OMELET

	Ingredients	1 Portion	2 Portions
Protein	Egg whites	4 whites	8 whites
	Ham, low-sodium, chopped	½ cup	1 cup
Veggie	Onion, chopped	2 Tbsp	4 Tbsp
	Green bell pepper, chopped	2 Tbsp	4 Tbsp

Follow directions for The Basic Omelet above.

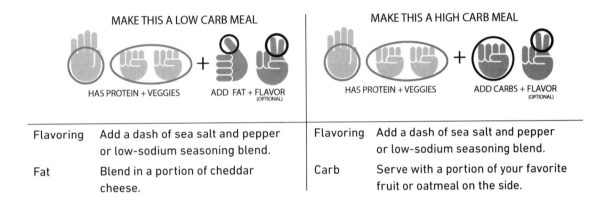

Flavoring	Add a dash of sea salt and pepper or low-sodium seasoning blend.	Flavoring	Add a dash of sea salt and pepper or low-sodium seasoning blend.
Fat	Blend in a portion of cheddar cheese.	Carb	Serve with a portion of your favorite fruit or oatmeal on the side.

SOUTHWESTERN OMELET

	Ingredients	1 Portion	2 Portions
Protein	Egg whites	3 whites	6 whites
	Ham, low-sodium, chopped	2 Tbsp	4 Tbsp
	Onion, chopped	1 Tbsp	2 Tbsp
Veggie	Green bell pepper, chopped	1 Tbsp	2 Tbsp
	Tomato, diced	1 Tbsp	2 Tbsp
	Salsa, fresh	1 Tbsp	2 Tbsp

Follow directions for The Basic Omelet above.

MAKE THIS A LOW CARB MEAL	MAKE THIS A HIGH CARB MEAL
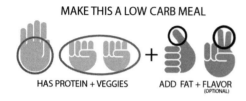	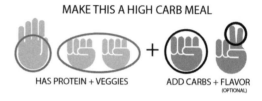
HAS PROTEIN + VEGGIES ADD FAT + FLAVOR (OPTIONAL)	HAS PROTEIN + VEGGIES ADD CARBS + FLAVOR (OPTIONAL)

Fat	Blend in a portion of cheddar cheese.	Carb	Omit cheese and serve with your favorite fruit, whole grain toast, or oatmeal on the side
Flavoring	Add a dash of sea salt and pepper or low-sodium seasoning blend.	Flavoring	Add a dash of sea salt and pepper or low-sodium seasoning blend.

BREAKFAST BURRITO

	Ingredients	1 Portion	2 Portions
Protein	Egg whites	3 whites	6 whites
	Ground turkey	2 Tbsp	4 Tbsp
Veggie	Baby spinach	1 handful	2 handfuls
	Romaine lettuce	1–2 leaves	2–4 leaves
Flavoring	Fresh salsa	1 Tbsp	2 Tbsp

1. Spritz cooking spray in a medium nonstick pan over medium heat. Add turkey and cook through. Set aside.
2. In a large bowl, whisk egg whites for about 45 seconds.
3. In another nonstick pan over medium-high heat, spritz cooking spray. Add the egg mixture to the pan. As the egg starts to set, add turkey and baby spinach and scramble until cooked.
4. Wrap the turkey-egg-spinach mixture in one or two leaves of romaine lettuce. Spoon the salsa over the top, then roll up and enjoy!

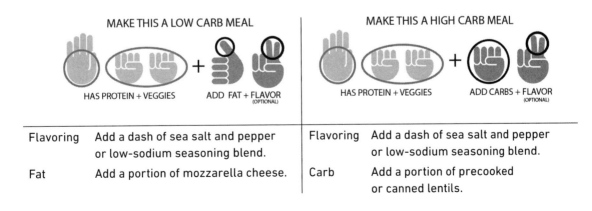

	MAKE THIS A LOW CARB MEAL		MAKE THIS A HIGH CARB MEAL
	HAS PROTEIN + VEGGIES · ADD FAT + FLAVOR (OPTIONAL)		HAS PROTEIN + VEGGIES · ADD CARBS + FLAVOR (OPTIONAL)
Flavoring	Add a dash of sea salt and pepper or low-sodium seasoning blend.	Flavoring	Add a dash of sea salt and pepper or low-sodium seasoning blend.
Fat	Sprinkle a portion of shredded cheddar cheese over the top of the burrito.	Carb	Wrap the whole burrito in a whole grain tortilla, brown rice tortilla, or two corn tortillas.

GREEN CHILE SCRAMBLE

	Ingredients	1 Portion	2 Portions
Protein	Egg whites	4 whites	8 whites
Veggie	Mushrooms, sliced	½ cup	1 cup
	Onion, chopped	1 Tbsp	2 Tbsp
	Green chilies, chopped	½ Tbsp	1 Tbsp

1. In a large bowl, whisk together egg whites for about 45 seconds.
2. Spritz cooking spray in a medium nonstick pan over medium-high heat. Add the egg mixture to the pan. As the egg starts to set, add mushrooms, onion, and green chilies. Scramble until cooked to taste. Enjoy!

	MAKE THIS A LOW CARB MEAL		MAKE THIS A HIGH CARB MEAL
	HAS PROTEIN + VEGGIES · ADD FAT + FLAVOR (OPTIONAL)		HAS PROTEIN + VEGGIES · ADD CARBS + FLAVOR (OPTIONAL)
Flavoring	Add a dash of sea salt and pepper or low-sodium seasoning blend.	Flavoring	Add a dash of sea salt and pepper or low-sodium seasoning blend.
Fat	Add a portion of mozzarella cheese.	Carb	Add a portion of precooked or canned lentils.

EGG MUFFIN SANDWICH (HIGH-CARB DAYS ONLY!)

	Ingredients	1 Portion	2 Portions
Protein	Egg whites	4 whites	8 whites
Veggie	Tomato, sliced	2 slices	4 slices
Carb	Ezekiel 4:9 brand English muffin, toasted	1	2

1. In a large bowl, whisk together egg whites for about 45 seconds.
2. Spritz cooking spray in a medium nonstick pan over medium-high heat. Add the egg mixture to the pan. As the egg starts to set, scramble until cooked.
3. Place the sliced tomato and cooked eggs on the muffin and enjoy!

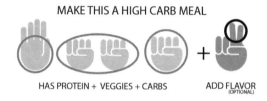

MAKE THIS A HIGH CARB MEAL

HAS PROTEIN + VEGGIES + CARBS   ADD FLAVOR (OPTIONAL)

Flavoring	Add a dash of sea salt and pepper or low-sodium seasoning blend.

COTTAGE CHEESE DESSERT

	Ingredients	1 Portion	2 Portions
Protein	Low-fat cottage cheese	½ cup	1 cup
Veggie	Celery sticks (stalks cut into 4–5- x ⅓–½-inch sticks)	4–5 sticks	8–10 sticks
Flavoring	SweetLeaf flavored stevia drops (berry, orange vanilla, banana, cinnamon, etc.)	1–5 drops	1–5 drops

1. Place cottage cheese in a bowl and add SweetLeaf flavored stevia drops to taste.
2. Enjoy with celery on the side.

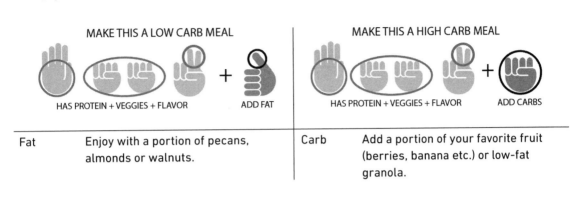

	MAKE THIS A LOW CARB MEAL		MAKE THIS A HIGH CARB MEAL
Fat	Enjoy with a portion of pecans, almonds or walnuts.	Carb	Add a portion of your favorite fruit (berries, banana etc.) or low-fat granola.

SONORAN COTTAGE CHEESE

	Ingredients	1 Portion	2 Portions
Protein	Low-fat cottage cheese	½ cup	1 cup
Veggie	Tomato, chopped	¼ cup	½ cup
Flavoring	Salsa, fresh	2 Tbsp	4 Tbsp

In a bowl, stir cottage cheese, salsa, and chopped tomato together. Enjoy!

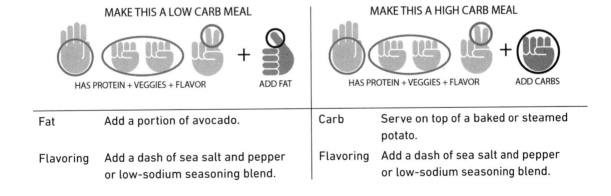

	MAKE THIS A LOW CARB MEAL		MAKE THIS A HIGH CARB MEAL
Fat	Add a portion of avocado.	Carb	Serve on top of a baked or steamed potato.
Flavoring	Add a dash of sea salt and pepper or low-sodium seasoning blend.	Flavoring	Add a dash of sea salt and pepper or low-sodium seasoning blend.

GREEK YOGURT PARFAIT

	Ingredients	1 Portion	2 Portions
Protein	Nonfat Plain Greek Yogurt	¾ cup	1½ cups
Veggie	Celery sticks (stalks cut into 4–5- x ⅓-½-inch sticks)	4–5 sticks	8–10 sticks
Flavoring	SweetLeaf flavored stevia drops (berry, orange, vanilla, banana, cinnamon, etc.)	1–5 drops	1–5 drops

1. Place yogurt in a bowl and add flavored stevia drops to taste.
2. Enjoy with celery on the side.

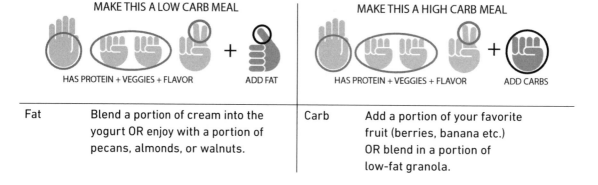

MAKE THIS A LOW CARB MEAL — HAS PROTEIN + VEGGIES + FLAVOR + ADD FAT

MAKE THIS A HIGH CARB MEAL — HAS PROTEIN + VEGGIES + FLAVOR + ADD CARBS

Fat	Blend a portion of cream into the yogurt OR enjoy with a portion of pecans, almonds, or walnuts.	Carb	Add a portion of your favorite fruit (berries, banana etc.) OR blend in a portion of low-fat granola.

TOMATO, BASIL, AND GARLIC CHICKEN

	Ingredients	2 Portions	4 Portions	6 Portions	8 Portions
Protein	Chicken breasts	2 breasts	4 breasts	6 breasts	8 breasts
Prep	Olive oil in spritzer bottle	1 spritz	2 spritzes	3 spritzes	4 spritzes
Flavoring	Tomato, basil and garlic seasoning (Mrs. Dash has a good one!)	2 tsp	4 tsp	6 tsp	8 tsp

1. Sprinkle the seasoning over both sides of chicken breasts.
2. Heat oil in a nonstick pan over medium heat. Add chicken breasts; cook on each side until done to your taste.
3. Serve immediately with your favorite side for a high- or low-carb day; or portion out and store in the fridge or freezer until you're ready to reheat and enjoy.

MAKE THIS A LOW CARB MEAL	MAKE THIS A HIGH CARB MEAL
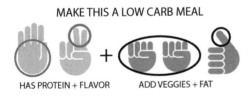	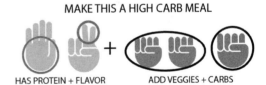
HAS PROTEIN + FLAVOR ADD VEGGIES + FAT	HAS PROTEIN + FLAVOR ADD VEGGIES + CARBS

Veggie	Serve with sliced tomatoes and baby spinach sprinkled with the tomato, basil, and garlic seasoning.	Veggie	Serve with a side salad or veggies of your choosing.
Fat	Drizzle a portion of olive oil over tomatoes and spinach.	Carb	Serve with your favorite carb side dish, such as baked potato, brown rice, or quinoa.
Flavoring	Add a drizzle of balsamic vinegar.		

CARIBBEAN JERK CHICKEN

	Ingredients	2 Portions	4 Portions	6 Portions	8 Portions
Protein	Chicken breasts	2	4	6	8
Prep	Olive oil in spritzer bottle	1 spritz	2 spritzes	3 spritzes	4 spritzes
Flavoring	Soy sauce, low-sodium	2 tsp	4 tsp	2 Tbsp	2½ Tbsp
	Cider vinegar	1 tsp	2 tsp	1 Tbsp	4 tsp
	Caribbean jerk seasoning	1 Tbsp	2 Tbsp	3 Tbsp	4 Tbsp
	Water	1 tsp	2 tsp	1 Tbsp	4 tsp

1. Put all ingredients into a gallon-size zip-top bag and seal. Gently massage bag to mix ingredients and fully coat meat with marinade. Let sit for at least 30 minutes (see do-ahead tip box!).

2. Remove meat from bag and discard any remaining marinade. Grill over medium heat or broil, cooking on each side to desired doneness.

3. Serve immediately with your favorite side for a high- or low-carb day; or portion out and store in the fridge or freezer until you're ready to reheat and enjoy.

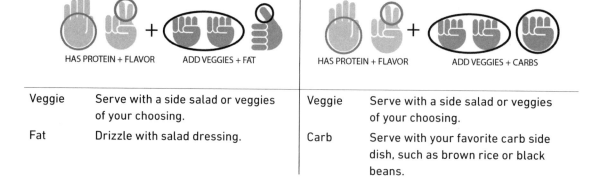

MAKE THIS A LOW CARB MEAL		MAKE THIS A HIGH CARB MEAL	
HAS PROTEIN + FLAVOR ADD VEGGIES + FAT		HAS PROTEIN + FLAVOR ADD VEGGIES + CARBS	
Veggie	Serve with a side salad or veggies of your choosing.	Veggie	Serve with a side salad or veggies of your choosing.
Fat	Drizzle with salad dressing.	Carb	Serve with your favorite carb side dish, such as brown rice or black beans.

Do-Ahead Tip: When your recipe calls for a marinade, marinate your ingredients the night before or on the morning of cooking to speed up dinnertime. It'll add even more flavor to your meat!

ITALIAN HERBED CHICKEN

	Ingredients	2 Portions	4 Portions	6 Portions	8 Portions
Protein	Chicken breasts	2	4	6	8
Prep	Olive oil in spritzer bottle	1 spritz	2 spritzes	3 spritzes	4 spritzes
Flavoring	Dried red pepper, ground	Dash	⅛ tsp	¼ tsp	⅜ tsp
	Garlic powder	⅛ tsp	¼ tsp	½ tsp	¾ tsp
	Seasoned salt	⅓ tsp	⅔ tsp	1 tsp	1⅓ tsp
	Italian seasoning	½ tsp	1 tsp	1½ tsp	2 tsp
	Red wine vinegar	4 tsp	2½ Tbsp	4 Tbsp	5½ Tbsp
	Water	1 tsp	2 tsp	1 Tbsp	4 tsp

1. Put all ingredients in a gallon-size zip-top bag and seal. Gently massage bag to mix ingredients and fully coat meat with marinade. Let sit for at least 30 minutes (see do-ahead tip box on page 216!).

2. Remove meat from bag and discard any remaining marinade. Grill over medium-high heat or broil, cooking on each side to desired doneness.

3. Serve immediately with your favorite side for a high- or low-carb day; or portion out and store in the fridge or freezer until you're ready to reheat and enjoy.

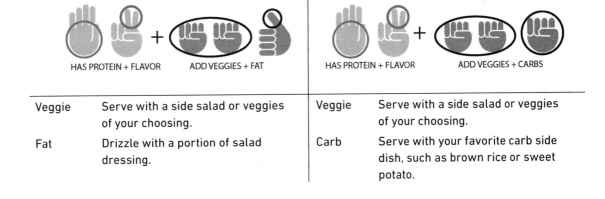

Veggie	Serve with a side salad or veggies of your choosing.	Veggie	Serve with a side salad or veggies of your choosing.
Fat	Drizzle with a portion of salad dressing.	Carb	Serve with your favorite carb side dish, such as brown rice or sweet potato.

LEMON CHICKEN

	Ingredients	2 Portions	4 Portions	6 Portions	8 Portions
Protein	Chicken breast	2	4	6	8
Prep	Olive oil in spritzer bottle	1 spritz	2 spritzes	3 spritzes	4 spritzes
Flavoring	Lemon juice	¼ cup	½ cup	¾ cup	1 cup
	Garlic, minced	1 tsp	2 tsp	1 Tbsp	4 tsp
	Salt and pepper to taste				

1. Put all ingredients in a gallon-size zip-top bag and seal. Gently massage bag to mix ingredients and fully coat meat with marinade. Let sit for at least 30 minutes (see do ahead tip box on page 216!).

2. Remove meat from bag and discard any remaining marinade. Broil, or grill over medium-high heat, cooking chicken on each side to desired doneness.

3. Serve immediately with your favorite side for a high- or low-carb day; or portion out and store in the fridge or freezer until you're ready to reheat and enjoy.

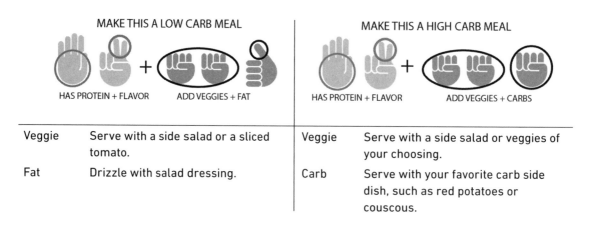

MAKE THIS A LOW CARB MEAL		MAKE THIS A HIGH CARB MEAL	
HAS PROTEIN + FLAVOR	ADD VEGGIES + FAT	HAS PROTEIN + FLAVOR	ADD VEGGIES + CARBS
Veggie	Serve with a side salad or a sliced tomato.	**Veggie**	Serve with a side salad or veggies of your choosing.
Fat	Drizzle with salad dressing.	**Carb**	Serve with your favorite carb side dish, such as red potatoes or couscous.

APPLE CIDER CHICKEN
(HIGH-CARB DAYS ONLY!)

	Ingredients	2 Portions	4 Portions	6 Portions	8 Portions
Protein	Chicken breasts	1½ breasts	3 breasts	4½ breasts	6 breasts
	Turkey bacon slices, diced	2 slices	4 slices	6 slices	8 slices
Prep	Olive oil in spritzer bottle	1 spritz	2 spritzes	3 spritzes	4 spritzes
	Butter*	1 tsp	2 tsp	1 Tbsp	4 tsp
Carb	Apple, cored and diced	¼ cup	½ cup	¾ cup	1 cup
	Apple cider	2 Tbsp	¼ cup	½ cup	¾ cup
	Brown rice	1 cup	2 cups	3 cups	4 cups
Flavoring	Chicken broth, low-sodium	2 Tbsp	¼ cup	½ cup	¾ cup
	Thyme, dried	½ tsp	1 tsp	1½ tsp	2 tsp
	Salt and pepper to taste				

*While butter is a fat, it's in such a small amount in this recipe that it's considered incidental and categorized as a prep food.

1. Heat oil in a nonstick pan over medium heat. Add chicken breasts and season to taste with salt and pepper. Cook on each side until done to your taste.
2. Remove chicken from pan and keep warm.
3. Add turkey bacon to the pan and cook for 4 to 5 minutes, until it is browned. Add apple and thyme; season with salt and pepper to taste.
4. As apples turn soft and start to brown, add cider and chicken broth. Increase the heat to medium-high. Cook until the sauce thickens, stirring frequently.
5. Add butter and stir until melted. Return the chicken to the pan, coating in sauce, and heat for 2 to 3 minutes. Serve immediately over brown rice, or portion out and store in the fridge or freezer until you're ready to reheat and enjoy.

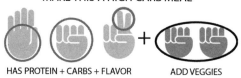

Veggie	Serve with either a spring-mix salad and sautéed onions or your favorite steamed veggies, such as broccoli or asparagus.

CHICKEN RATATOUILLE

	Ingredients	2 Portions	4 Portions	6 Portions	8 Portions
Protein	Chicken breasts	2	4	6	8
Prep	Olive oil in spritzer bottle	1 spritz	2 spritzes	3 spritzes	4 spritzes
Veggie	Green bell pepper, cut into strips	½ cup	1 cup	1½ cups	2 cups
	Onion, diced	½ cup	1 cup	1½ cups	2 cups
	Eggplant, diced	½ cup	1 cup	1½ cups	2 cups
	Zucchini, sliced	½ cup	1 cup	1½ cup	2 cups
	14-oz can diced tomatoes with garlic	½ can	1 can	1½ cans	2 cans
	Baby spinach	2 cups	4 cups	6 cups	8 cups

1. Heat oil in a nonstick pan over medium heat. Add meat and green pepper strips and stir frequently, until chicken is almost done.

2. Add the onion, eggplant, and zucchini and stir frequently, until veggies are tender (about 3 minutes).

3. Stir in tomatoes and bring to a boil. Reduce heat and simmer until heated through.

4. To serve: Place about 1 cup of spinach on each plate. Spoon the ratatouille over the top of the spinach; the heat will wilt the spinach. Top off with parmesan cheese if desired.

5. To store: Portion out ratatouille and store in the fridge or freezer until ready to reheat, then serve over spinach leaves as above.

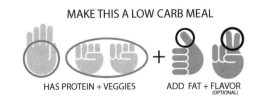

MAKE THIS A LOW CARB MEAL

HAS PROTEIN + VEGGIES   ADD FAT + FLAVOR (OPTIONAL)

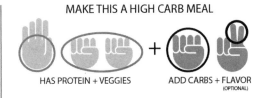

MAKE THIS A HIGH CARB MEAL

HAS PROTEIN + VEGGIES   ADD CARBS + FLAVOR (OPTIONAL)

| Fat | Add a portion of grated parmesan or mozzarella cheese | Carb | Serve over couscous. |

BUFFALO-GARLIC TURKEY BURGERS

	Ingredients	2 Portions	4 Portions	6 Portions	8 Portions
Protein	Ground turkey	8 oz raw	16 oz raw	24 oz. raw	32 oz raw
Prep	Olive oil in spritzer bottle	1 spritz	2 spritzes	3 spritzes	4 spritzes
Flavoring	Garlic, minced	1 tsp	2 tsp	1 Tbsp	4 tsp
	Cayenne pepper	¼ tsp	½ tsp	¾ tsp	1 tsp
	Hot sauce (optional)	½ tsp	1 tsp	1½ tsp	2 tsp

1. Place the ground turkey in a bowl and sprinkle it with the cayenne pepper and garlic. Add hot sauce if desired. Knead, mixing turkey and seasoning. Form into patties.
2. Heat oil in a nonstick pan over medium heat. Add patties and cook on each side until done to your taste.
3. Place turkey patties on a plate.
4. Serve immediately with your favorite side for a high- or low-carb day; or portion out and store in the fridge or freezer until you're ready to reheat and enjoy.

MAKE THIS A LOW CARB MEAL		MAKE THIS A HIGH CARB MEAL	

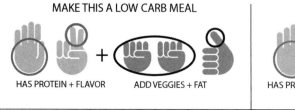

| HAS PROTEIN + FLAVOR | ADD VEGGIES + FAT |

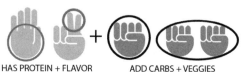

| HAS PROTEIN + FLAVOR | ADD CARBS + VEGGIES |

Fat	Top turkey patty with a portion of your favorite cheese. I like pepperjack!	Carb	Add a baked sweet potato or boiled red potatoes on the side.
Veggie	Serve with celery sticks, carrot sticks, and/or raw broccoli.	Veggie	Serve with celery sticks, carrot sticks, and/or raw broccoli.

CITRUS STEAK

	Ingredients	2 Portions	4 Portions	6 Portions	8 Portions
Protein	Sirloin steak, boneless and lean	6 oz	12 oz	18 oz	24 oz
Prep	Olive oil in spritzer bottle	1 spritz	2 spritzes	3 spritzes	4 spritzes
Flavoring	Orange juice	1 Tbsp	2 Tbsp	3 Tbsp	4 Tbsp
	Lime juice	2 tsp	4 tsp	6 tsp	8 tsp
	Steak seasoning	2 tsp	4 tsp	6 tsp	8 tsp
	Dried oregano	½ tsp	1 tsp	1½ tsp	2 tsp
	Cumin, ground	⅛ tsp	¼ tsp	½ tsp	¾ tsp
Veggie	Onion, sliced (optional)	1	2	3	4

1. Put all ingredients except onions in a gallon-size zip-top bag and seal. Gently massage bag to mix ingredients and fully coat meat with marinade. Let sit for at least 30 minutes (see do-ahead tip box on page 216).
2. While the meat is marinating, grill the onion slices to your liking (if desired).
3. Grill steak over medium-high heat, cooking on each side until desired doneness.

4. Serve immediately with onions (if desired), a baked potato or baked sweet potato, and a side salad or vegetable for a high-carb day, or portion out and store in the fridge or freezer until you're ready to reheat and enjoy.

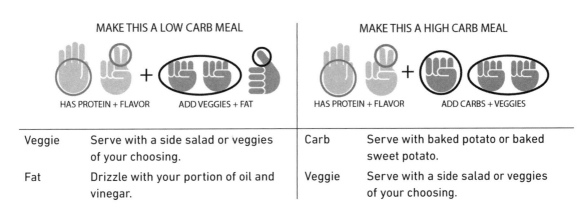

MAKE THIS A LOW CARB MEAL		MAKE THIS A HIGH CARB MEAL	
HAS PROTEIN + FLAVOR / ADD VEGGIES + FAT		HAS PROTEIN + FLAVOR / ADD CARBS + VEGGIES	
Veggie	Serve with a side salad or veggies of your choosing.	Carb	Serve with baked potato or baked sweet potato.
Fat	Drizzle with your portion of oil and vinegar.	Veggie	Serve with a side salad or veggies of your choosing.

ROSEMARY STEAK TENDERLOIN

	Ingredients	2 Portions	4 Portions	6 Portions	8 Portions
Protein	Sirloin steak, boneless and lean	6 oz	12 oz	18 oz	24 oz
Prep	Olive oil spray	1 spritz	2 spritzes	3 spritzes	4 spritzes
Flavoring	Steak seasoning	¾ tsp	1½ tsp	2¼ tsp	1 Tbsp
	Parsley flakes	1 tsp	2 tsp	1 Tbsp	4 tsp
	Rosemary flakes	1 tsp	2 tsp	1 Tbsp	4 tsp

1. Spritz each steak with olive oil spray.
2. Sprinkle the steaks with steak seasoning, parsley, and rosemary.
3. Grill over high heat or broil, cooking on each side to desired doneness.
4. Serve immediately with your favorite side for a high- or low-carb day; or portion out and store in the fridge or freezer until you're ready to reheat and enjoy.

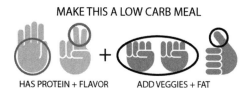

MAKE THIS A LOW CARB MEAL	MAKE THIS A HIGH CARB MEAL
HAS PROTEIN + FLAVOR ADD VEGGIES + FAT	HAS PROTEIN + FLAVOR ADD VEGGIES + CARBS

Veggie	Serve with a side salad or veggies of your choosing.	Veggie	Serve with a side salad or veggies of your choosing.
Fat	Drizzle with salad dressing.	Carb	Serve with your favorite carb side dish, such as brown rice or sweet potato.

ROASTED GARLIC BEEF-AND-VEGGIE STIR-FRY

	Ingredients	2 Portions	4 Portions	6 Portions	8 Portions
Protein	Sirloin steak, boneless and lean	6 oz	12 oz	18 oz	24 oz
Prep	Olive oil in spritzer bottle	1 spritz	2 spritzes	3 spritzes	4 spritzes
Flavoring	Soy sauce, low-sodium	2 tsp	4 tsp	6 tsp	8 tsp
	Cornstarch	½ tsp	1⅓ tsp	2 tsp	2⅔ tsp
	Ginger, ground	⅛ tsp	¼ tsp	½ tsp	¾ tsp
	Roasted garlic and bell pepper seasoning	1 tsp	2 tsp	3 tsp	4 tsp
Veggie	Assorted veggies, including broccoli florets, bell pepper strips, and snow peas	2 cups	4 cups	6 cups	8 cups
	Water	⅓ cup	⅔ cup	1 cup	1⅓ cups

1. Cut steak into ¼-inch strips.
2. In a small bowl, mix together soy sauce, cornstarch, ginger, roasted garlic and bell pepper seasoning, and water. Set aside.
3. Heat oil in a large nonstick pan over medium-high heat. Add sliced beef in small batches and cook until no longer pink (about 5 minutes). Remove from pan and repeat until all meat is cooked.

4. If needed, spritz the pan with a bit more oil. Add the veggies and cook for 3 to 4 minutes, stirring frequently.

5. Add the meat to the veggies and stir in the soy sauce mixture. Continue stirring while the liquid comes to a boil. Simmer for about a minute more.

6. Serve immediately; or portion out and store in the fridge or freezer until you're ready to reheat and enjoy.

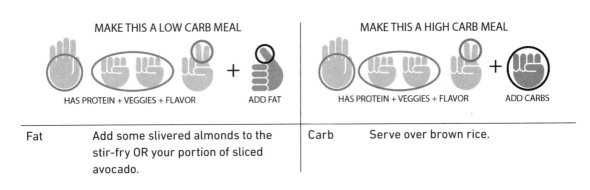

	MAKE THIS A LOW CARB MEAL		MAKE THIS A HIGH CARB MEAL	
Fat	Add some slivered almonds to the stir-fry OR your portion of sliced avocado.		Carb	Serve over brown rice.

BLUE CHEESE CUBE STEAK (LOW-CARB DAYS ONLY!)

	Ingredients	2 Portions	4 Portions	6 Portions	8 Portions
Protein	Cube steak	6 oz	12 oz	18 oz	24 oz
Fat	Blue cheese crumbles	1/3 cup	2/3 cup	1 cup	1 1/3 cup
Prep	Olive oil in spritzer bottle	1 spritz	2 spritzes	3 spritzes	4 spritzes
Flavoring	Red onion, finely chopped	1/2 Tbsp	1 Tbsp	1 1/2 Tbsp	2 Tbsp
	Salt and pepper to taste				

1. Turn on oven broiler to preheat.

2. On stovetop, heat oil in a nonstick pan over medium heat. Add steaks; cook on each side until done to your taste.

3. Place steaks on broiler pan lined with foil (for easy cleaning!) and top each steak with blue cheese and onion.

4. Broil steaks just until cheese is melted.

5. Serve immediately with your favorite side for a low-carb day.

6. To store: After removing meat from stove, portion it out and store in the fridge or freezer until you're ready to use it. Separately, portion out onion and blue cheese and store in fridge or freezer until you're ready to use it. To cook, follow steps 3 through 5 OR place steaks in microwaveable container, top with blue cheese and onion, and cook in microwave.

MAKE THIS A HIGH CARB MEAL

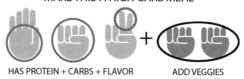

HAS PROTEIN + CARBS + FLAVOR   ADD VEGGIES

Veggie   Serve with steamed broccoli or asparagus.

SIRLOIN STEAK WITH GREEN BEANS AND TOMATOES

	Ingredients	2 Portions	4 Portions	6 Portions	8 Portions
Protein	Sirloin steak, boneless and lean	6 oz	12 oz	18 oz	24 oz
Prep	Olive oil in spritzer bottle	1 spritz	2 spritzes	3 spritzes	4 spritzes
Veggie	Green beans	1 cup (2 handfuls)	2 cups (4 handfuls)	3 cups (6 handfuls)	4 cups (8 handfuls)
	Tomatoes, chopped into large pieces	1 tomato	2 tomatoes	3 tomatoes	4 tomatoes
Flavoring	Garlic, minced	¾ tsp	1½ tsp	2¼ tsp	1 Tbsp
	Salt and pepper to taste				

1. Heat oil in a nonstick pan on high heat. Add meat; cook on each side to desired doneness. Remove from pan and keep warm.

2. Lower heat to medium. Add green beans and sauté for about 3 minutes; add garlic and continue cooking for about a minute. Season with salt and pepper to taste.

3. Add diced tomatoes to the pan and cook for about a minute. Cover pan and cook for an additional 3 to 4 minutes, until tomatoes become somewhat saucy.

4. Plate the meat with vegetables on the side. Serve immediately with your favorite side for a high- or low-carb day; or portion out and store in the fridge or freezer until you're ready to reheat and enjoy. Green beans and tomatoes can be refrigerated but will not freeze well.

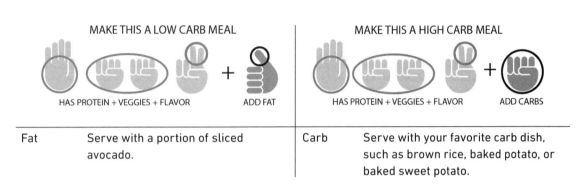

Fat	Serve with a portion of sliced avocado.	Carb	Serve with your favorite carb dish, such as brown rice, baked potato, or baked sweet potato.

HONEY-VANILLA GLAZED PORK TENDERLOIN

	Ingredients	2 Portions	4 Portions	6 Portions	8 Portions
Protein	Pork Tenderloin, lean	6 oz	12 oz	18 oz	24 oz
Flavoring	Honey	1 Tbsp	2 Tbsp	3 Tbsp	¼ cup
	Vinegar	½ Tbsp	1 Tbsp	1½ Tbsp	2 Tbsp
	Vanilla	¼ tsp	½ tsp	¾ tsp	1 tsp
	Paprika	⅛ tsp	¼ tsp	⅜ tsp	½ tsp
	Ground mustard	Dash	⅛ tsp	¼ tsp	⅜ tsp
	Salt and pepper to taste				

*While honey is a carb and has an impact on blood sugar, the amount used here is so minimal it is considered incidental and counted as a flavoring.

1. In a zip-top bag, combine honey and flavorings. Close and knead bag to mix ingredients.
2. Add pork tenderloins and knead to cover each with the glaze.
3. Heat a nonstick pan over medium heat. Add pork tenderloins; cook on each side until done to your taste.
4. Serve immediately with your favorite side salad or vegetable; or portion out and store in the fridge or freezer until you're ready to reheat and enjoy.

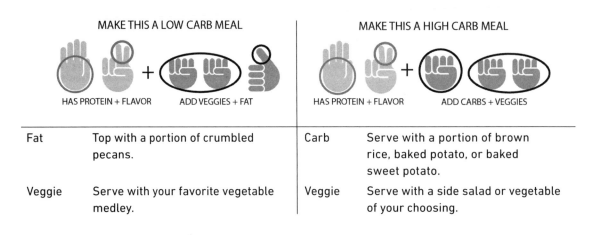

MAKE THIS A LOW CARB MEAL		MAKE THIS A HIGH CARB MEAL	
HAS PROTEIN + FLAVOR	ADD VEGGIES + FAT	HAS PROTEIN + FLAVOR	ADD CARBS + VEGGIES
Fat	Top with a portion of crumbled pecans.	Carb	Serve with a portion of brown rice, baked potato, or baked sweet potato.
Veggie	Serve with your favorite vegetable medley.	Veggie	Serve with a side salad or vegetable of your choosing.

MOM'S HERBED PORK DINNER

	Ingredients	2 Portions	4 Portions	6 Portions	8 Portions
Protein	Pork tenderloins, lean	6 oz	12 oz	18 oz	24 oz
Prep	Olive oil in spritzer bottle	1 spritz	2 spritzes	3 spritzes	4 spritzes
Flavoring	Paprika	½ tsp	1 tsp	1½ tsp	2 tsp
	Thyme, dried	¼ tsp	½ tsp	¾ tsp	1 tsp
	Salt	¼ tsp	½ tsp	¾ tsp	1 tsp
	Black pepper	⅛ tsp	¼ tsp	½ tsp	¾ tsp

1. Mix flavorings in a bowl. Sprinkle evenly over tenderloins.

2. Heat oil in a nonstick pan over medium heat. Add pork tenderloins; cook on each side until done to your taste.

3. Serve immediately with your favorite side salad or vegetable; or portion out and store in the fridge or freezer until you're ready to reheat and enjoy.

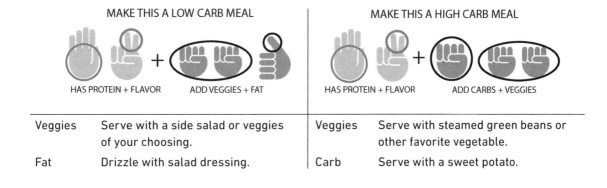

MAKE THIS A LOW CARB MEAL		MAKE THIS A HIGH CARB MEAL	
HAS PROTEIN + FLAVOR	ADD VEGGIES + FAT	HAS PROTEIN + FLAVOR	ADD CARBS + VEGGIES
Veggies	Serve with a side salad or veggies of your choosing.	Veggies	Serve with steamed green beans or other favorite vegetable.
Fat	Drizzle with salad dressing.	Carb	Serve with a sweet potato.

ROASTED-GARLIC-AND-HERB PORK

	Ingredients	2 Portions	4 Portions	6 Portions	8 Portions
Protein	Pork tenderloins, lean	6 oz	12 oz	18 oz	24 oz
Prep	Olive oil in spritzer bottle	1 spritz	2 spritzes	3 spritzes	4 spritzes
Flavoring	Roasted-garlic-and-herb seasoning	2 tsp	4 tsp	6 tsp	8 tsp

1. Sprinkle seasoning over pork tenderloins.

2. Heat oil in a nonstick pan on medium heat. Add pork tenderloins; cook on each side until done to your taste.

3. Serve immediately with your favorite side for a high- or low-carb day; or portion out and store in the fridge or freezer until you're ready to reheat and enjoy.

MAKE THIS A LOW CARB MEAL	MAKE THIS A HIGH CARB MEAL

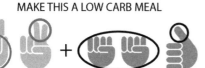
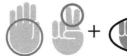
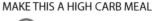
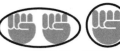

HAS PROTEIN + FLAVOR   ADD VEGGIES + FAT   HAS PROTEIN + FLAVOR   ADD VEGGIES + CARBS

Veggies	Serve with a side salad sprinkled with the roasted-garlic-and-herb seasoning.	Veggies	Serve with steamed asparagus or other favorite vegetable.
Fat	Drizzle greens with a little olive oil and balsamic vinegar and toss to serve.	Carb	Serve with a portion of brown rice.

SPICED PAPRIKA PORK

	Ingredients	2 Portions	4 Portions	6 Portions	8 Portions
Protein	Pork tenderloin, lean	6 oz	12 oz	18 oz	24 oz
Prep	Butter*	1 tsp	2 tsp	1 Tbsp	4 tsp
	Olive oil in spritzer bottle	1 spritz	2 spritzes	3 spritzes	4 spritzes
Flavoring	Paprika	½ tsp	1 tsp	1½ tsp	2 tsp
	Oregano, dried	¼ tsp	½ tsp	¾ tsp	1 tsp
	Cumin, ground	½ tsp	1 tsp	1½ tsp	2 tsp
	Garlic powder	½ tsp	1 tsp	1½ tsp	2 tsp
	Salt	¼ tsp	½ tsp	¾ tsp	1 tsp
	Fennel seeds	⅛ tsp	¼ tsp	½ tsp	¾ tsp
	Cayenne pepper, ground	Dash	⅛ tsp	¼ tsp	⅜ tsp
	Chicken broth	¼ cup	½ cup	¾ cup	1 cup

*While butter is a fat, it's used in such a small amount in this recipe that it's considered incidental and categorized as a prep food.

1. In small bowl, combine all of the spices.
2. Sprinkle half of the spice mixture over one side of each pork tenderloin.
3. Heat oil in a nonstick pan over medium heat. Add pork, spiced side down. While it's cooking, sprinkle the tops with the remaining spice mix.

4. Continue cooking until browned on the first side, then turn and continue cooking until done to your taste.
5. Remove tenderloins from pan and keep warm.
6. Add butter to the pan and whisk up all the browned spices and bits. Turn heat up to medium-high. Add chicken broth and continue whisking until sauce reduces by about half.
7. Plate pork tenderloins and drizzle sauce over the top. Serve immediately with your favorite side for a high- or low-carb day; or portion out and store in the fridge or freezer until you're ready to reheat and enjoy. Portion out sauce mix separately in snack-size zip-top bags.

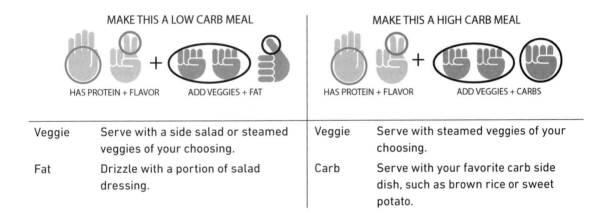

	MAKE THIS A LOW CARB MEAL		MAKE THIS A HIGH CARB MEAL
Veggie	Serve with a side salad or steamed veggies of your choosing.	Veggie	Serve with steamed veggies of your choosing.
Fat	Drizzle with a portion of salad dressing.	Carb	Serve with your favorite carb side dish, such as brown rice or sweet potato.

CARIBBEAN PORK TENDERLOIN

	Ingredients	2 Portions	4 Portions	6 Portions	8 Portions
Protein	Pork tenderloin, lean	6 oz	12 oz	18 oz	24 oz
Prep	Olive oil in spritzer bottle	1 spritz	2 spritzes	3 spritzes	4 spritzes
Flavoring	Caribbean jerk seasoning	½ Tbsp	1 Tbsp	1½ Tbsp	2 Tbsp

1. Sprinkle seasoning over both sides of the pork tenderloins.
2. Heat oil in a nonstick pan over medium heat. Add pork tenderloins; cook on each side until done to your taste.

3. Serve immediately with your favorite side for a high- or low-carb day; or portion out and store in the fridge or freezer until you're ready to reheat and enjoy.

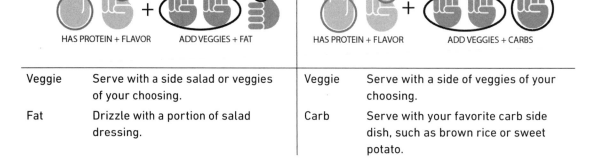

MAKE THIS A LOW CARB MEAL		MAKE THIS A HIGH CARB MEAL	
HAS PROTEIN + FLAVOR	ADD VEGGIES + FAT	HAS PROTEIN + FLAVOR	ADD VEGGIES + CARBS
Veggie	Serve with a side salad or veggies of your choosing.	Veggie	Serve with a side of veggies of your choosing.
Fat	Drizzle with a portion of salad dressing.	Carb	Serve with your favorite carb side dish, such as brown rice or sweet potato.

ITALIAN GARLIC-AND-HERB SHRIMP SALAD

	Ingredients	2 Portions	4 Portions	6 Portions	8 Portions
Protein	Large raw shrimp, peeled and deveined	25 shrimp	50 shrimp	75 shrimp	100 shrimp
Prep	Olive oil in spritzer bottle	1 spritz	2 spritzes	3 spritzes	4 spritzes
Flavoring	Roasted garlic-and-herb seasoning	2 tsp	4 tsp	2 Tbsp	2 Tbsp + 2 tsp

1. Sprinkle seasoning over the raw shrimp, turning to ensure they're evenly coated.
2. Heat oil in a nonstick pan over medium heat. Add shrimp; stir frequently until shrimp are cooked.
3. Serve immediately; or portion out shrimp and store in the fridge or freezer until you're ready to reheat and enjoy.

MAKE THIS A LOW CARB MEAL		MAKE THIS A HIGH CARB MEAL	

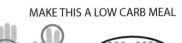
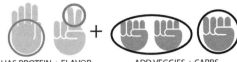

| | HAS PROTEIN + FLAVOR | ADD VEGGIES + FAT | | HAS PROTEIN + FLAVOR | ADD VEGGIES + CARBS |

Veggie	Serve over a bed of raw baby spinach.	Veggie	Serve over a bed of raw baby spinach.
Fat	Drizzle a little olive oil and balsamic vinegar over the spinach and toss before topping with shrimp.	Carb	Serve with your favorite carb side dish, such as brown rice, red potatoes, or sweet potato.

CHIPOTLE-LIME HALIBUT (OR TILAPIA)

	Ingredients	2 Portions	4 Portions	6 Portions	8 Portions
Protein	Halibut or tilapia filets	8 oz	16 oz	24 oz	32 oz
Prep	Olive oil	½ Tbsp	1 Tbsp	1½ Tbsp	2 Tbsp
Flavoring	Cilantro, fresh chopped	½ tsp	1 tsp	1½ tsp	2 tsp
	McCormick Grill Mates Chipotle Pepper Marinade	¼ package	½ package	¾ package	1 package
	Lime juice	½ Tbsp	1 Tbsp	1½ Tbsp	2 Tbsp
	Water	1 Tbsp	2 Tbsp	3 Tbsp	¼ cup

Tip: Many fish recipes can be prepared with different fish.

1. In a zip-top bag, combine marinade, oil, water, lime juice, and cilantro. Close and knead bag to mix ingredients.
2. Add fish to bag and turn bag over several times to cover evenly with the marinade. Refrigerate for at least 15 minutes.
3. Preheat grill or broiler. Remove fish from bag and discard remaining marinade. Grill over medium heat or broil on each side until done to your taste. (It cooks quickly, so keep an eye on it!)

4. Serve immediately with your favorite side for high- or low-carb day; or portion out fish and store in fridge up to 2 to 3 days. (Not recommended for freezing.) When you're ready to eat, reheat and enjoy.

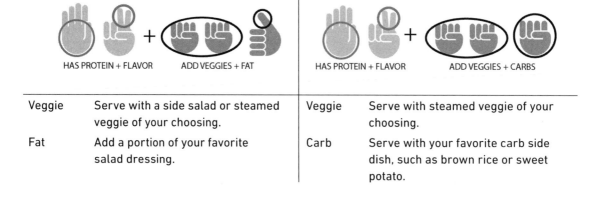

MAKE THIS A LOW CARB MEAL		MAKE THIS A HIGH CARB MEAL	
Veggie	Serve with a side salad or steamed veggie of your choosing.	Veggie	Serve with steamed veggie of your choosing.
Fat	Add a portion of your favorite salad dressing.	Carb	Serve with your favorite carb side dish, such as brown rice or sweet potato.

CAJUN SALMON

	Ingredients	2 Portions	4 Portions	6 Portions	8 Portions
Protein	Salmon filets	8 oz	16 oz	24 oz	32 oz
Fat	Butter*	½ Tbsp	1 Tbsp	1½ Tbsp	2 Tbsp
Flavoring	Cajun seasoning	1 Tbsp	2 Tbsp	3 Tbsp	4 Tbsp
	Garlic, minced	1 tsp	2 tsp	1 Tbsp	4 tsp
	Balsamic vinegar	2 Tbsp	¼ cup	¼ cup	¾ cup
	Lemon wedges	2	4	6	8

*While butter is a fat, it's in such a small amount in this recipe that it's considered incidental and categorized as a prep food.

1. Heat half the butter in a nonstick pan over medium heat. Add salmon; cook on each side until almost done. (It cooks quickly, so keep an eye on it!)
2. Remove salmon from pan and keep warm.
3. Add remaining butter along with the garlic and the Cajun seasoning. Cook for about 2 minutes.

4. Add balsamic vinegar to pan and cook for an additional 2 minutes, stirring constantly.

5. Return the salmon to the pan and finish cooking. Plate each filet with a lemon wedge.

6. Serve immediately; or portion out and store in the fridge up to 2 to 3 days. (Not recommended for freezing.) When you're ready to eat, reheat and enjoy.

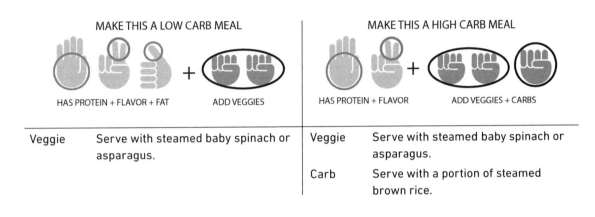

MAKE THIS A LOW CARB MEAL		MAKE THIS A HIGH CARB MEAL	
Veggie	Serve with steamed baby spinach or asparagus.	Veggie	Serve with steamed baby spinach or asparagus.
		Carb	Serve with a portion of steamed brown rice.

CREAMY HORSERADISH SALMON (LOW-CARB DAYS ONLY!)

	Ingredients	2 Portions	4 Portions	6 Portions	8 Portions
Protein	Salmon filet	8 oz	16 oz	24 oz	32 oz
Prep	Olive oil spray	1 spritz	2 spritzes	3 spritzes	4 spritzes
Flavoring	Basil, dried	¼ tsp	½ tsp	¾ tsp	1 tsp
	Garlic powder	¼ tsp	½ tsp	¾ tsp	1 tsp
Fat	Sour cream	¼ cup	½ cup	¾ cup	1 cup
	Mayonnaise	½ Tbsp	1 Tbsp	1½ Tbsp	2 Tbsp
Flavoring	Horseradish sauce	½ Tbsp	1 Tbsp	1½ Tbsp	2 Tbsp
	Salt and pepper to taste				

1. Mix sour cream, mayonnaise, and horseradish sauce in a small bowl.

2. Heat oil in a nonstick pan over medium heat. Sprinkle one side of fish with basil, garlic powder, salt, and pepper. Place fish in pan, seasoned side down. Sprinkle the top of the fish with the remaining seasoning. Turn when nicely browned on one side and continue cooking on the other side until done to your taste.

3. Plate fish and garnish each serving with a thumb-size dollop of horse-radish cream. Serve immediately; or portion out fish and sauce separately and store in the fridge up to 2 to 3 days. (Not recommended for freezing.) When you're ready to eat, reheat and enjoy.

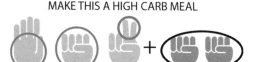

MAKE THIS A HIGH CARB MEAL

HAS PROTEIN + CARBS + FLAVOR   ADD VEGGIES

Veggies	Serve with a side of steamed asparagus or broccoli.

GINGER-LIME SALMON

	Ingredients	2 Portions	4 Portions	6 Portions	8 Portions
Protein	Salmon filets	8 oz	16 oz	24 oz	32 oz
Carb	Honey*	½ Tbsp	1 Tbsp	1½ Tbsp	2 Tbsp
Flavoring	Ginger root, grated	2 tsp	4 tsp	6 tsp	8 tsp
	Garlic, minced	1 tsp	2 tsp	1 Tbsp	4 tsp
	Soy sauce, low-sodium	½ Tbsp	1 Tbsp	1½ Tbsp	2 Tbsp
	Lime juice	2 Tbsp	¼ cup	½ cup	¾ cup
	Green onions (scallions), chopped	1 Tbsp	2 Tbsp	3 Tbsp	4 Tbsp

*While honey is a carb and has an impact on blood sugar, the amount used in this recipe is so minimal that it's considered incidental and counted as a flavoring.

1. Put half of the green onions, plus the honey, ginger, garlic, soy sauce, and lime juice, in a gallon-size zip-top bag and seal. Gently massage bag to mix ingredients and then add fish, turning bag over several times to fully coat with marinade. Let sit for at least 30 minutes (see do ahead tip box on page 216).

2. Remove fish from bag and discard any remaining marinade. Place fish on a broiler pan (line with aluminum foil for easy cleaning!). Broil under medium-high heat until cooked through.

3. Plate fish and garnish with remaining green onions. Serve immediately or portion out and store in fridge up to 2 to 3 days. (Not recommended for freezing.) When you're ready to eat, reheat and enjoy.

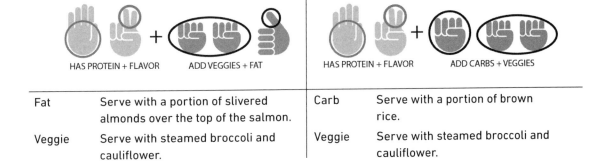

MAKE THIS A LOW CARB MEAL — HAS PROTEIN + FLAVOR + ADD VEGGIES + FAT

MAKE THIS A HIGH CARB MEAL — HAS PROTEIN + FLAVOR + ADD CARBS + VEGGIES

Fat	Serve with a portion of slivered almonds over the top of the salmon.		Carb	Serve with a portion of brown rice.
Veggie	Serve with steamed broccoli and cauliflower.		Veggie	Serve with steamed broccoli and cauliflower.

APPENDIX A

CARB-CYCLING FAQS

THE CYCLE

What's Carb Cycling?

Essentially, it's a weight-loss system designed to keep your metabolism as high as possible so you can burn fat like crazy! It's laid out in *one-week segments* that alternate days of high-carbohydrate eating with days of low-carbohydrate eating. On high-carb days, your meals are higher in carbs and slightly higher in calories, and on low-carb days your meals (except breakfast) are almost entirely carb-free and slightly lower in calories. Carb cycling keeps your protein intake constant from meal to meal and day to day, and on low-carb days you can eat certain fats!

Each week, you repeat your carb-cycling pattern. The net result is a wonderfully balanced nutrition program that keeps your metabolism stoked up in order to *melt away maximum fat!* High-carb days boost your metabolism, which then stays high on low-carb days, burning more fat than it would on a static or stable nutrition program that has you eating the same way every day.

The basic carb-cycling pattern is simple: You eat a high-carb diet every other day and a low-carb diet on the days in between. But you can alternate high-carb and low-carb days in *various ways*, depending on your weight-loss goals. In this book, I give you four different cycles: one for slow and easy weight loss, one for fast weight loss, one for superfast weight loss, and one for weight loss combined with maximum athletic performance.

Some cycles have more high-carb days and some have more low-carb days than the basic cycle.

Why Do I Have to Eat Five Meals a Day?

You need to eat healthy food five times a day to feed your metabolism when it cycles on every three hours. Adding fuel makes the fire burn hotter and incinerate fat faster. The more you eat, the more you lose! You want that, right?

At first, you'll feel like you're eating too much, because you'll be eating a lot of bulk. The real, whole, healthy foods in the carb-cycling diet are high in fiber—that's the bulk—and low in calories. They keep you fuller longer, so when mealtime rolls around every three hours, you might not even be hungry! Eat anyway, and eat the types and amounts of food that I ask you to. Don't worry, you'll adjust quickly!

What Are Reward Days and Reward Meals?

One day a week, or several meals per week, you take a *reward day or meal*. These are days or meals that you select to indulge in the foods you crave, even if they are unhealthy. (See Appendix C for a list of some reward food options.) Rewarding yourself like this keeps your cravings from going haywire and throwing you off your carb-cycling course. It's also a way to reward yourself for sticking to your carb-cycling program. It's absolutely *necessary* to reward yourself at least once a week!

What's a Slingshot?

A Slingshot is seven high-carb days in a row. But isn't carb cycling about alternating high-carb and low-carb days? It sure is, but sooner or later your body's going to adapt to your cycle and slow down its fat burning. To keep your weight loss from plateauing, you'll be doing a one-week Slingshot after every three weeks of carb cycling. It's an essential part of carb cycling.

When you stop carb cycling for a week to load your body with carbs, your body will feel all that fuel flowing in and crank up your metabolism to its hottest! If you've reached a weight-loss plateau, your fat-burning system will reboot and your carb-cycling machine will be up and running again. If you haven't plateaued, the Slingshot will retune your carb-cycling engine so it keeps purring along.

What Are Shredders?

They're cardiovascular workouts that I've designed especially for carb cyclers like you. Aerobic activities like walking, bicycling, jumping rope, and hiking get your metabolism firing to its maximum fat-burning level. That's why I also call Shredder workouts *accelerators*. You do your Shredders five days a week, for as little as five minutes if you're just starting to carb cycle, and as much as sixty minutes if you're far along on your weight-loss journey.

What Are Shapers?

These are workouts that shape and develop your muscles—muscle-building exercise that some people call resistance training or strength training. Using the most fundamental movements of the human body—running, jumping, pushing, pulling, crunching, and squatting—these brief, vigorous workouts jack up your metabolism by building your muscles, the biggest energy consumers in your body. You'll do them first thing in the morning, five days a week, to rev up your metabolism for the rest of the day.

What Are 9-Minute Missions?

For this book, I've created a set of twenty new Shapers I call 9-Minute Missions. Focusing on different parts of your body, each one can be completed in nine minutes and will inject some variety into your workout. Try them out and you'll never get bored of sculpting your muscles and burning fat!

The Food

What Should I Do About All the Unhealthy Food in My Kitchen?

It's there in your home, your office, your car, your secret hiding places: food that'll sabotage your weight-loss mission. You love that stuff, but there's no way around it. You *must* toss anything unhealthy—sugary, fatty, salty, processed, refined, fast, and junk food—that makes your mouth water. Don't worry: You can always eat the bad stuff when it's time for a reward day or meal. But the rest of the time, you'll only succeed with carb cycling if you create a temptation-free environment for success. Some of the sabotage junk foods that you should chuck might surprise you; others are no-brainers. Here's a partial list:

- Alcoholic beverages: beer, wine, and hard liquor
- Baked goods such as bagels, white bread, cake, cookies, crackers, pretzels, donuts, and pastries
- Candy
- Chips
- Chocolate
- Fried food
- Frozen dishes and meals
- Fruit juice
- Ice cream
- Soda with sugar

You must also get rid of *all* foods containing the following ingredients:

- Brown sugar
- Corn syrup
- Hydrogenated oils
- Raw sugar
- White flour
- White rice
- White sugar

What About Artificial Sweeteners?

Most sugar-free foods and diet drinks are sweetened with *artificial ingredients* such as saccharin (Sweet'N Low), sucralose (Splenda), and aspartame (Equal, NutraSweet). They can be useful while you're cutting back on sugary processed food and getting used to eating whole, healthy food. But artificial sweeteners are chemicals, and the jury's still out on whether they have any health impacts. *Natural sweeteners* like stevia (e.g., SweetLeaf, Truvia), xylitol (e.g., Xlear, XyloSweet), and sorbitol (used in many chewing gums, toothpastes, and other products) come from plant sources and are very low in calories. It may be a good idea to eventually switch from artificial sweeteners to natural sweeteners.

How Can I Save Money When I Eat Healthy?

First off, you're going to discover that eating healthy is actually less expensive than eating your old way. I keep my body full of healthy food for only a few dollars a day! How do I do it? Two words: bulk food. By purchasing healthy food in bulk online and at your local discount warehouse stores (Costco, Sam's Club, etc.), you can enjoy big savings. To find your nearest warehouse store, or to find bulk-food websites, just do a quick online search. Then hop in the car or click on the URL, and you'll be well on your way to cheap, nutritious eating. Feed your body what it really wants! (Note: The quantities given below are for one person.)

Buy online:

- Whole grains, beans, and lentils (you can buy either dried or canned beans and lentils, but the dried varieties are less expensive): A three-month supply runs about $25.
- Protein powder (our main protein source): Three-months' worth costs about $90. This comes out to about 20 cents per scoop, which means you get two to five shakes for only a dollar!

Buy at warehouse stores:

- Frozen cruciferous vegetables (e.g., cauliflower, cabbage, bok choy, and broccoli): A two-week supply is around $15.
- Poultry (especially chicken breasts; frozen is cheaper): You can get a week's supply for about $15.
- Root vegetables: Enough for two weeks = $10, more or less.
- Frozen and fresh fruits and vegetables: For two weeks' worth, you'll pay around $20.
- Flavors and seasonings (e.g., garlic, onions, spices, and dried herbs): The cost of these is just pennies per serving!

What Are the Best Food-Prep Tools for Carb Cycling?

I've found these to be the most useful:

- Blender
- George Foreman electric grill
- Japanese-style electric rice cooker
- Shaker bottles for making protein shakes
- Toaster oven
- Veggie steamer

- Food scale
- Measuring cups and spoons
- Food storage containers

Why Should I Prepare My Food in Bulk?

Preparing your food in bulk, *hours or days ahead* of when you'll be eating it, helps guarantee your carb-cycling success! To maintain your weight-loss lifestyle, you have to eat the right foods at the right time of day, starting with breakfast within thirty minutes of getting up and then eating every three hours, for a total of five meals a day.

Most of us can't prepare our food every three hours, so to make sure you eat right, you've got to have your meals *ready and waiting.* The best way to do this is to prepare several days' worth of food a couple times a week. I recommend that you prep in bulk every three to four days—you won't have to cook for the rest of the week! Right after you prepare it, portion your food into containers and refrigerate it. Prepping your food in bulk preps you for long-term success!

The Process

Are Before and After Pictures a Good Idea?

Yes! Pictures are *proof of your progress* and success—they can keep you going when you're discouraged and they're a great *reality check* when your body image gets distorted. With all the physical changes and emotional ups and downs you're experiencing, your eyes will sometimes play tricks on you: What you see in the mirror is *not* reality. Here are five photo pointers:

1. Remember that these pics are just for you! Nobody else has to see them unless you want to share.

2. Take pictures no more than once a week. You can see your progress on a day-to-day basis, but when you line up your weekly pictures, you will be amazed by your transformation!

3. This might be scary at first: Wear clothing that gives you a full view of your body, so you can really see where and how you're transforming. Shorts (and for women, a sports bra) are a good bet.

4. Snap photos from a few different angles—at least a front shot and a side/profile shot. Your body will be changing in a lot of different ways, and you don't want to miss anything!

5. Use your pics for daily motivation. Stick them up in places where your eyes frequently land. Inside your fridge, on your bathroom mirror, next to your bed, or at the bottom of a drawer you use a lot are all good spots. To really kick your butt, use them as your screen saver!

How Can I Maximize My Carb-Cycling Results?

It's *completely normal* for your weight loss to lag a little now and then. The Slingshot (see the FAQ above) takes care of this on a higher level, but on the daily level you can use some simple techniques to keep your carb cycling in top form:

- Drink at least a gallon of water a day.
- Make sure to eat breakfast every day, within thirty minutes of waking up.
- Make sure to eat every three hours.
- Watch your portions. Use the portioning and calorie chart in Chapter 6, "Feed Your Fire: The Recipes," to bring your meals into line with carb-cycling requirements.
- Keep an eye on your reward eating so you don't overdo it. See Appendix C, "Reward Foods," for sample calorie counts.

How Can I Control My Cravings?

We all have cravings, and you're going to run up against them while you're transitioning to your new, healthy lifestyle. The key is to manage your cravings. A few tips:

- Drink at least one tall glass of water when a craving starts. It's easy to confuse thirst with hunger, so stay hydrated!
- Chew sugar-free mint-flavored gum, eat a sugar-free breath mint, or put a dab of toothpaste on your tongue. The mint flavor suppresses your appetite so you can make it to the next meal without cheating.
- Eat high-fiber foods and add volume to your meals with veggies galore! Fiber-rich food stays in your stomach and small intestine longer, keeping you full. This technique is especially effective early in the day: Eating plenty of fiber at breakfast helps suppress your appetite for the rest of the day.
- On your low-carb days, when you're more likely to crave carbs, have a little fat! Eat one tablespoon of your favorite healthy fat (e.g. almond butter), set your timer for fifteen minutes, and bam! Your sweet and salty cravings will disappear.

When Should I Weigh Myself?

The fluctuating numbers that you see on your scale from day to day don't reveal anything about your overall weight loss: Your body weight naturally varies because of water retention and flushing and other factors. As a gauge of your weight change, your scale will give you a meaningful number only every week or two. Weigh in only once a week to see an informative figure (see the chart on page 92 for more information). We have a tendency to rely on our weight as a measure of our success, but other changes in your body are actually more accurate. See the next FAQ.

How Can I Tell My Body Is Changing?

Not surprisingly, the first tool dieters turn to is their bathroom scale. It's a great tool, but pounds aren't the only measure of weight loss—and they don't give you the whole picture. Some other signs that you're on the right track toward losing weight are:

- Clothing: The way your clothes fit is the *best* gauge of your progress.
- Inches: Decreasing waist, hip, thigh, and neck dimensions show you *where* you're slimming down.
- Appetite: Your hunger level will fluctuate as you switch between high- and low-carb days because you're getting more fuel (= less hunger) on high days and less fuel (= more hunger) on low days. Feeling your metabolic tank fill up and empty out is a sign that carb cycling's doing what it should!
- Cravings: On low-carb days, when your body's getting few carbs, it's natural to have more food cravings—*of course you want more calories!* Cravings aren't as much of a problem on high-carb days—though they don't totally disappear—because your body's getting plenty of calories. Yes! You're carb cycling!
- Energy level: You'll feel an energy surge on high-carb days and a drop in your energy level on low-carb days.
- Mental clarity: On low-carb days you might be a little slower as your brain gets fewer carbs. This shows that your carb cycle's in action.
- Water retention and flushing: This is another reason *not* to rely only on the scale. Your weight is higher after high-carb days because your body is retaining water; on low-carb days the water will flush out and your weight will drop. Your numbers might go up four pounds one day and drop five pounds the next, rise two pounds then fall three pounds—you get the picture. What those numbers *really* prove is that your carb cycling is going well.
- Body temperature: Lots of fuel on high-carb days makes your metabolism burn hot, and your temperature might rise slightly. You may find

yourself stripping the blankets off the bed. The opposite can happen on low-carb, low-fuel days. It's your carb cycle at work!

Why Am I Losing Inches but Not Pounds?

When you first start carb cycling—even for a couple of weeks—the number on your scale might not budge. But at the same time, you might be losing inches, and your clothing size might be shrinking. Confusing, isn't it? You're experiencing *recomposition*, adding muscle mass while subtracting fat, so your net weight stays the same. Once your body gets used to your new nutrition and exercise regime, muscle growth will slow down and you'll burn fat faster. Voilà! You're losing weight!

APPENDIX B

EASY NO-PREP FOODS

Sometimes, you just need a completely hassle-free meal, and sometimes, you might run out of the food you've prepared ahead of time—oops! Well, you've got plenty of options for fueling up without having to do any prep. Because they can be ready to go anywhere, anytime, no-prep foods are especially handy when you're *traveling*. Just swing by a grocery store when you reach your destination and pick up a few convenient items. Here are a few of my recommendations:

Protein

- **Powdered and liquid protein (whey, egg, soy, and vegetable):** These are the easiest to use and the *least expensive* source for your daily protein requirements: You can substitute them for any other protein in your meal plan! Can't find chicken, fish, or beef soon enough? Protein powder/shakes save the day! Available in *many different flavors*, protein drinks kind of taste like milk shakes. It's easy to carry them with you anywhere! Pop open a can or mix a scoop of powder with water, and you've got an instant meal. You can drink your protein, and it won't leave you feeling too full. Be sure to pick a powder that is 100 percent protein with no (or low/incidental) carbs and fat.

- **Meal Replacement Shakes:** These are one of the easiest, tastiest, and most convenient ways to get an instant and nutritious meal. They are already a combination of protein, carbs, fiber, vitamins, and minerals. Just add water or milk, shake, and enjoy!

- **Cottage cheese and yogurt:** Two other sources of quick and convenient protein that you can often take with you. You've got to keep them refrigerated, but when you're ready to eat, you *just open the container.* Eat your cottage cheese plain, season it with salt and pepper, sweeten it with stevia, or mix in some no-prep fruit on high-carb days (bananas, grapes, berries, orange, or tangerine segments). Choose low-sugar, low- or nonfat yogurt; avoid the kind with sugary fruit preserves already in the container. Greek yogurt is a great pick. If you want fruit in your yogurt, mix in the no-prep fruits mentioned above.

- **Low-sodium canned fish and meat:** Here's a speedy, trouble-free way to include fish, chicken, and beef in your recipes. The quality and nutritional value aren't quite as good as the fresh version, but you can use them *the second you open the can.* Just beware: Sodium content can be extremely high in canned foods.

- **Low-sodium deli meat:** Sliced turkey breast, chicken breast, and roast beef from the deli are ready to go anytime, though they do require refrigeration. Ask for the thickest, freshest cuts, and *avoid the pre-packaged kinds!*

Carbohydrates

- **Fruit:** Large fruits, like apples and oranges, are already packaged in the right portions. You have to measure out berries, cherries, and grapes and put them in a plastic bag or container, but that takes only a minute or so. Fruit's super-portable!

- **Low-fat, low-sugar cereal:** Bran cereal and granola are packed with high-fiber whole grain. They're perfect for snacking and are great for traveling.

- **Ezekiel 4:9 brand products:** You can find this brand of hearty bread, made from sprouted grains, in the health food freezer at your supermarket. It comes in the form of loaves, wraps, and pita pockets, and there are also different flavors of breakfast cereal.

- **Low-sodium canned legumes (beans and lentils):** A fast and simple source of complex carbs and protein. Just open the can and heat them up! They're best if you *flavor them up* with spices, herbs, or hot sauce.

- **Yams and sweet potatoes:** Poke a few holes in their skin with a fork or knife, wrap them in a wet paper towel, and pop 'em into the microwave for a few minutes. If you buy the right size (about 4 inches long and 2.5 inches in diameter is nearly 100 calories), *each one is a perfect portion!* You can even take cooked yams and sweet potatoes with you on the go and eat them at room temperature.

- **Dry oatmeal:** Portion it out and *blend it into your protein shake* for a hearty, delicious combo of carbs and protein.

Vegetables

- **Frozen Veggies:** Pop 'em in the microwave for a couple of minutes and they're ready to go!

- **Raw veggies:** You can eat a lot of vegetables raw. Broccoli, carrots, celery, cucumbers, peppers, radishes, sprouts, tomatoes, and zucchini make great snacks—and you can *eat as much as you want!* Cut 'em up and pop them into a plastic bag or container to take with you anywhere. Some veggies even come cleaned and cut, so you have even less to do.

- **Bagged salads:** These are generally pre-cleaned, so you can just open the bag, grab as much as you want, and munch! *Ignore the little bags of premade dressing* and use a nice vinaigrette or other low-fat dressing.

Fats

- **Cheese:** The *right kind* of cheese (see the list of recommended foods in Chapter 6, "Feed Your Fire: The Recipes") is a great source of healthy fat. The string and pre-sliced forms are perfectly portioned, and string cheese makes a tasty snack on the road.

- **Almond and peanut butters:** These are two of my favorites: One tablespoon of the good old-fashioned stuff—*the kind with the oil on top*, which you mix in—has about a hundred calories and always hits the spot. It's an excellent choice when you need to rein in carb cravings.

- **Pecans, almonds, and walnuts:** The healthiest of the nuts, these are delicious both roasted and raw. Go for *plain or lightly salted* versions: Smokehouse and other flavored varieties are loaded with sodium and sugar! Portion your nuts into plastic bags or containers for a terrific traveling snack.

- **Avocados:** Rich in healthy fats, these are wonderful on their own (I like a dash of salt) and are good complements to protein, carbs, and veggies alike! Peel, cut, and eat.

- **Salad dressing:** It's easy to add zest to a salad—or other veggies—with a little dressing. The bottled kinds sold at your supermarket are mega-convenient, but make sure to avoid sugary and sweet varieties. If you're into creamy dressing, buy the low-fat kind. Vinaigrettes are usually the healthiest choice.

APPENDIX C

REWARD FOODS

Finally, your reward day or reward meal has arrived. You're psyched for a taste of your favorite foods. What to eat? How much? I give you your freedom with that, but it's a good idea to watch what you're doing. With rewards come responsibilities: Before you scarf down that ice cream or tear open that bag of chips, read the nutritional information label and find out how many calories you're getting. When you're planning a night out at a chain restaurant, visit the chain's website for the calorie counts of the food they serve. Here are some reward foods and their typical calorie counts. And remember, a lot of reward foods are loaded with sodium, so you may see the number on the scale jump for a few days afterward!

SAMPLE REWARD FOOD SERVINGS AND CALORIE COUNTS		
Food	Serving Size	Calories
Cheeseburger, basic	average fast-food size	500
Hot dog	1 regular-length dog, with bun	370
French fries	average fast-food serving	350
Sandwich cookies	3 cookies	160
Pepperoni pizza	1 slice of a 14-inch pie	350
Soda	12 oz	150
Chicken tenders	3 tenders	350

(continued on next page)

SAMPLE REWARD FOOD SERVINGS AND CALORIE COUNTS		
Food	Serving Size	Calories
Vanilla ice cream	4-oz scoop	260
Glazed donut	1 donut	260
Potato chips	1-oz bag	160
Cheesecake	small slice, about 3½ oz	350
Caramel-nut-chocolate candy bar	2-oz bar	271
Barbecue Buffalo wings	6 wings	600
Macaroni and cheese	side portion, about 8 oz	300
Baby-back barbecue ribs	approx. 1 lb	563
Chocolate chip cookie	large cookie, about 2 oz	380
Oatmeal-raisin cookie	large cookie, about 2 oz	235
Lasagna	lunch portion, about 4 inches square	600
Chocolate milkshake	16 oz	420
Nachos supreme	7 oz	430

MULTIPLE-SERVING MEASUREMENT CHART

The recipes in Chapter 6, "Feed Your Fire: The Recipes," include ingredient measurements that yield either one, two, four, six, or eight servings of each dish. Whether you want to make larger quantities to freeze and eat later or you plan to serve more than two people at a meal, you will, of course, need to use more ingredients. But you can use lots of recipes that aren't in Chapter 6, including the ones in my first book, *Choose to Lose*, and others that you find in different sources or make up yourself. You won't have multiple-serving measurements for any of those, so you've got to figure out, say, how to turn a two-person recipe into one that serves eight, or an eight-person recipe into one that serves two. You could do the math yourself, but here's a chart that makes multiplying and dividing your recipes a whole lot easier.

Note: Where the table gives oddball quantities, such as ⅛, ⅓, or ⅜ tsp or ½ Tbsp, just do your best to eyeball the amount in the next-larger measuring spoon. Fill a tablespoon halfway for ½ Tbsp, fill a half-teaspoon a little below the rim for ⅓ tsp, and so on.

MEASUREMENT CONVERSIONS FOR MULTIPLYING RECIPES

2 Servings	4 Servings	6 Servings	8 Servings
Dash	⅛ tsp	¼ tsp	⅜ tsp
⅛ tsp	¼ tsp	⅜ tsp	½ tsp
¼ tsp	½ tsp	¾ tsp	1 tsp
⅓ tsp	⅔ tsp	1 tsp	1⅓ tsp
½ tsp	1 tsp	1½ tsp	2 tsp
¾ tsp	1½ tsp	2¼ tsp	1 Tbsp
1 tsp	2 tsp	3 tsp (1 Tbsp)	4 tsp
½ Tbsp	1 Tbsp	1½ Tbsp	2 Tbsp
2 tsp	4 tsp	2 Tbsp	2 Tbsp + 2 tsp
1 Tbsp	2 Tbsp	3 Tbsp	¼ cup
1½ Tbsp	3 Tbsp	¼ cup + ½ Tbsp	⅜ cup
2 Tbsp	¼ cup	½ cup	¾ cup
¼ cup	½ cup	¾ cup	1 cup
⅓ cup	⅔ cup	1 cup	1⅓ cups
½ cup	1 cup	1½ cups	2 cups
⅔ cup	1⅓ cups	2 cups	2⅔ cups
¾ cup	1½ cups	2¼ cups	3 cups
1 cup	2 cups	3 cups	4 cups

9-MINUTE MISSION QUICK REFERENCE GUIDE

9 Minute Missions

Upper Body Missions

Push N Press	Crazy Eights	Drill Sergeant	Shoulder Shaker
Triangle Push Ups	8 Mountain Climber	Commander Push Ups	Bench Dip
Bench Dip	8 Bench Dip	Pike Press	Pike Press
Pike Press	8 Dive Bomber	Burpee	Squat Thrust

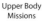

Core Missions

Hard Core	Easy Threezies	The Washboard	Lucky Thirteens
Swing Ups	3 Squat Thrusts	Mountain Climbers	13 Swing Ups
Knees to Elbows	6 Twisters	Swing Ups	13 Mountain Climbers
Mountain Climbers	9 Swing Ups	Plank	13 Twisters

Lower Body Missions

Thigh Master	Butt Out	Drop It Like Its Hot	Step It Up
Back Lunge	Squat Jacks	30 High Knees	Back Lunge
Air Squats	Marching Soldiers	20 Back Lunge	Bridge Ups
Bridge Ups	Back Lunge	10 Squat Jacks	Squat Jacks

Total Body Missions

Stack 'em Up	Run Like The Wind	Jackpot	Monday Funday
5 Squat Thrusts	High Knees	7 Twisters	Triangle Push Up
10 Swing Ups	Push Ups	7 Marching Soldiers	Twisters
15 Marching Soldiers	Back Lunge	7 Squat Thrusts	Air Squats

Five Alive	The Pulse Pounder	TGIF	Seven Eleven
5 Burpee	Burpee	Dive Bombers	11 Knees to Elbows
5 Twisters	Knees to Elbows	Knees to Elbows	7 Dive Bombers
5 Marching Soldiers	Air Squat	Air Squat	11 Mountain Climbers

FOUR-WEEK PERSONAL LOGS

EASY CYCLE
Sample Weeks

This week I promise to:

	Monday	Tuesday	Wednesday	Thursday	Friday	Saturday	Sunday
Wake Up	The clock starts as soon as you wake up. Eat breakfast within 30 minutes and meals are spaced every 3 hours thereafter.						
9-Minute Mission						Rest	Rest
Mission Type:	Stack 'em Up Super Circuits	Push n' Press Enduro	Hard Core Step Ladder	Thigh Master Sprinterval	Five Alive Rapid Rounds		
	I completed _____ circuits	_____ reps _____ reps _____ reps	I got up to _____ reps per circuit	_____ total reps _____ total reps _____ total reps	_____ rounds _____ rounds _____ rounds		

Shredders	Dirty Two-Thirties						
Intensity:	2min30sec low 2min30sec high	2min30sec low 2min30sec high	2min30sec low 2min30sec high	2min30sec low 2min30sec high	2min30sec low 2min30sec high	Rest	Rest
Overall Duration:	5 minutes	5 minutes	5 minutes	5 minutes	5 minutes		
Morning Weight:	X	X	X	X	X	Weigh In_____	X

MEAL TRACKER

	Monday	Tuesday	Wednesday	Thursday	Friday	Saturday	Sunday
	LC	HC 1	LC	HC 1	LC	HC 1	HC 1
Breakfast (within 30 min of waking)	PROTEIN + CARB	PROTEIN + CARB	PROTEIN + CARB	PROTEIN + CARB	PROTEIN + CARB	PROTEIN + CARB	PROTEIN + CARB
Morning Snack	PROTEIN + FAT	PROTEIN + CARB	PROTEIN + FAT	PROTEIN + CARB	PROTEIN + FAT	PROTEIN + CARB	REWARD MEAL 1
Lunch	PROTEIN + FAT	REWARD MEAL 1	PROTEIN + FAT	PROTEIN + CARB	PROTEIN + FAT	REWARD MEAL 1	PROTEIN + CARB
Afternoon Snack	PROTEIN + FAT	PROTEIN + CARB	PROTEIN + FAT	REWARD MEAL 1	PROTEIN + FAT	PROTEIN + CARB	PROTEIN + CARB
Dinner	PROTEIN + FAT	PROTEIN + CARB	PROTEIN + FAT	PROTEIN + CARB	PROTEIN + CARB	PROTEIN + CARB	PROTEIN + CARB

WATER INTAKE: ☐ 1/2 gallon (64 oz.) ☐ 1 gallon (128 oz.)

Drink 1 gallon (128 oz.) or at least half of your body weight in ounces of water. A 200lb person should drink at least 100 oz. of water.

WEEKLY REFLECTION

This week's accomplishments:

This week's challenges:

Strategies for next week:

Promises Broken?:

Confess to:
Reassess Promise(s):
Recommit:

This week I promise to:

	Monday	Tuesday	Wednesday	Thursday	Friday	Saturday	Sunday
Wake Up	The clock starts as soon as you wake up. Eat breakfast within 30 minutes and meals are spaced every 3 hours thereafter.						

9-Minute Mission

Mission Type:	Run Like The Wind Sprintervals	Crazy Eights Super Circuits	Easy Threezies Rapid Rounds	Butt Out Enduro	The Pulse Pounder Step Ladder	Rest	Rest
	_____total reps	I completed	_____rounds	_____reps	I got up to		
	_____total reps	_____circuits	_____rounds	_____reps	_____reps per circuit		
	_____total reps		_____rounds	_____reps			

Shredders			**Nasty Nineties**				
Intensity:	90 seconds low 90 seconds high	90 seconds low 90 seconds high	90 seconds low 90 seconds high	90 seconds low 90 seconds high	90 seconds low 90 seconds high	Rest	Rest
Overall Duration:	10 minutes	10 minutes	10 minutes	10 minutes	10 minutes		

Morning Weight:	X	X	X	X	X	Weigh In_____	X

MEAL TRACKER

	Monday	Tuesday	Wednesday	Thursday	Friday	Saturday	Sunday
	LC	HC 1	LC	HC 1	LC	HC 1	HC 1
Breakfast (within 30 min of waking)	PROTEIN + CARB	PROTEIN + CARB	PROTEIN + CARB	PROTEIN + CARB	PROTEIN + CARB	PROTEIN + CARB	PROTEIN + CARB
Morning Snack	PROTEIN + FAT	PROTEIN + CARB	PROTEIN + FAT	PROTEIN + CARB	PROTEIN + FAT	PROTEIN + CARB	REWARD MEAL
Lunch	PROTEIN + FAT	REWARD MEAL	PROTEIN + FAT	PROTEIN + CARB	PROTEIN + FAT	REWARD MEAL	PROTEIN + CARB
Afternoon Snack	PROTEIN + FAT	PROTEIN + CARB	PROTEIN + FAT	REWARD MEAL	PROTEIN + FAT	PROTEIN + CARB	PROTEIN + CARB
Dinner	PROTEIN + FAT	PROTEIN + CARB	PROTEIN + FAT	PROTEIN + CARB	PROTEIN + FAT	PROTEIN + CARB	PROTEIN + CARB

WATER INTAKE: ☐ 1/2 gallon (64 oz.)   ☐ 1 gallon (128 oz.)

Drink 1 gallon (128 oz.) or at least half of your body weight in ounces of water. A 200lb person should drink at least 100 oz. of water.

WEEKLY REFLECTION

This week's accomplishments:

This week's challenges:

Strategies for next week:

Promises Broken?:

Confess to:
Reassess Promise(s):
Recommit:

EASY CYCLE SAMPLE WEEK 3 of 4

This week I promise to:

	Monday	Tuesday	Wednesday	Thursday	Friday	Saturday	Sunday
Wake Up		The clock starts as soon as you wake up. Eat breakfast within 30 minutes and meals are spaced every 3 hours thereafter.					
9-Minute Mission						Rest	Rest
Mission Type:	Jackpot Rapid Rounds	Drill Sergeant Step Ladder	The Washboard Enduro	Drop It Like It's Hot Super Circuits	TGIF Sprintervals		
	_____ rounds	I got up to _____ reps per circuit	_____ reps	I completed _____ circuits	_____ total reps		
	_____ rounds		_____ reps		_____ total reps		
	_____ rounds		_____ reps		_____ total reps		

Shredders	Monday	Tuesday	**Mighty Minutes** Wednesday	Thursday	Friday	Saturday	Sunday
Intensity:	1 minute low 1 minute high	1 minute low 1 minute high	1 minute low 1 minute high	1 minute low 1 minute high	1 minute low 1 minute high	Rest	Rest
Overall Duration:	15 minutes	15 minutes	15 minutes	15 minutes	15 minutes		
Morning Weight:	X	X	X	X	X	Weigh In_____	X

MEAL TRACKER

	Monday	Tuesday	Wednesday	Thursday	Friday	Saturday	Sunday
	LC	HC 1	LC	HC 1	LC	HC 1	HC 1
Breakfast (within 30 min of waking)	PROTEIN + CARB	PROTEIN + CARB	PROTEIN + CARB	PROTEIN + CARB	PROTEIN + CARB	PROTEIN + CARB	PROTEIN + CARB
Morning Snack	PROTEIN + FAT	PROTEIN + CARB	PROTEIN + FAT	PROTEIN + CARB	PROTEIN + FAT	PROTEIN + CARB	1 REWARD MEAL
Lunch	PROTEIN + FAT	1 REWARD MEAL	PROTEIN + FAT	PROTEIN + CARB	PROTEIN + FAT	1 REWARD MEAL	PROTEIN + CARB
Afternoon Snack	PROTEIN + FAT	PROTEIN + CARB	PROTEIN + FAT	1 REWARD MEAL	PROTEIN + FAT	PROTEIN + CARB	PROTEIN + CARB
Dinner	PROTEIN + FAT	PROTEIN + CARB	PROTEIN + FAT	PROTEIN + CARB	PROTEIN + FAT	PROTEIN + CARB	PROTEIN + CARB

WATER INTAKE: ☐ 1/2 gallon (64 oz.)   ☐ 1 gallon (128 oz.)

Drink 1 gallon (128 oz.) or at least half of your body weight in ounces of water. A 200lb person should drink at least 100 oz. of water.

WEEKLY REFLECTION

This week's accomplishments:

This week's challenges:

Strategies for next week:

Promises Broken?:

Confess to:
Reassess Promise(s):
Recommit:

EASY CYCLE SAMPLE WEEK 4 of 4 - Slingshot Week

This week I promise to:

	Monday	Tuesday	Wednesday	Thursday	Friday	Saturday	Sunday
Wake Up	The clock starts as soon as you wake up. Eat breakfast within 30 minutes and meals are spaced every 3 hours thereafter.						
9-Minute Mission						Rest	Rest
Mission Type:	Monday Funday Enduro	Shoulder Shaker Sprintervals	Lucky Thirteen Super Circuits	Step It Up Step Ladder	Seven Eleven Rapid Rounds		
	_____reps _____reps _____reps	_____total reps _____total reps _____total reps	I completed _____ circuits	I got up to _____ reps per circuit	_____rounds _____rounds _____rounds		
Shredders		Thrilling Thirties					
Intensity:	30 seconds low 30 seconds high	30 seconds low 30 seconds high	30 seconds low 30 seconds high	30 seconds low 30 seconds high	30 seconds low 30 seconds high	Rest	Rest
Overall Duration:	20 minutes	20 minutes	20 minutes	20 minutes	20 minutes		
Morning Weight:	X	X	X	X	X	Weigh In_____	X

MEAL TRACKER

	Monday	Tuesday	Wednesday	Thursday	Friday	Saturday	Sunday
	HC 1	HC 1	HC 1	HC 1	HC 1	HC 1	HC 1
Breakfast (within 30 min of waking)	PROTEIN + CARB	PROTEIN + CARB	PROTEIN + CARB	PROTEIN + CARB	PROTEIN + CARB	PROTEIN + CARB	PROTEIN + CARB
Morning Snack	PROTEIN + CARB	PROTEIN + CARB	REWARD MEAL	PROTEIN + CARB	REWARD MEAL	PROTEIN + CARB	REWARD MEAL
Lunch	PROTEIN + CARB	REWARD MEAL	PROTEIN + CARB	PROTEIN + CARB	PROTEIN + CARB	REWARD MEAL	PROTEIN + CARB
Afternoon Snack	REWARD MEAL	PROTEIN + CARB	PROTEIN + CARB	REWARD MEAL	PROTEIN + CARB	PROTEIN + CARB	PROTEIN + CARB
Dinner	PROTEIN + CARB	PROTEIN + CARB	PROTEIN + CARB	PROTEIN + CARB	PROTEIN + CARB	PROTEIN + CARB	PROTEIN + CARB

WATER INTAKE: ☐ 1/2 gallon (64 oz.)   ☐ 1 gallon (128 oz.)

Drink 1 gallon (128 oz.) or at least half of your body weight in ounces of water. A 200lb person should drink at least 100 oz. of water.

WEEKLY REFLECTION

This week's accomplishments:

This week's challenges:

Strategies for next week:

Promises Broken?:

Confess to:
Reassess Promise(s):
Recommit:

For weeks 5-12 and beyond, follow the workout routines for the CLASSIC CYCLE.

CLASSIC CYCLE
Sample Weeks

CLASSIC CYCLE: SAMPLE WEEK 1 of 4

This week I promise to:

	Monday	Tuesday	Wednesday	Thursday	Friday	Saturday	Sunday
Wake Up	The clock starts as soon as you wake up. Eat breakfast within 30 minutes and meals are spaced every 3 hours thereafter.						

9-Minute Mission						Rest	Rest
Mission Type:	Stack 'em Up Super Circuit	Push n' Press Enduro	Hard Core Step Ladder	Thigh Master Sprinterval	Five Alive Rapid Rounds		
	I completed	_____reps	I got up to	_____total reps	_____rounds		
	_____	_____reps	_____reps	_____total reps	_____rounds		
	circuits	_____reps	per circuit	_____total reps	_____rounds		

Shredders	Dirty Two-Thirties						
Intensity:	2min30sec low 2min30sec high	2min30sec low 2min30sec high	2min30sec low 2min30sec high	2min30sec low 2min30sec high	2min30sec low 2min30sec high	Rest	Rest
Overall Duration:	5 minutes	5 minutes	5 minutes	5 minutes	5 minutes		

Morning Weight:	X	X	X	X	X	Weigh In_____	X

MEAL TRACKER

	Monday	Tuesday	Wednesday	Thursday	Friday	Saturday	Sunday
	LC	HC	LC	HC	LC	HC	★
Breakfast (within 30 min of waking)	PROTEIN + CARB	PROTEIN + CARB	PROTEIN + CARB	PROTEIN + CARB	PROTEIN + CARB	PROTEIN + CARB	Guilt Free Day
Morning Snack	PROTEIN + FAT	PROTEIN + CARB	PROTEIN + FAT	PROTEIN + CARB	PROTEIN + FAT	PROTEIN + CARB	Enjoy anything you'd like without overdoing it. Aim to intake about 1,000 more calories than normal.
Lunch	PROTEIN + FAT	PROTEIN + CARB	PROTEIN + FAT	PROTEIN + CARB	PROTEIN + FAT	PROTEIN + CARB	
Afternoon Snack	PROTEIN + FAT	PROTEIN + CARB	PROTEIN + FAT	PROTEIN + CARB	PROTEIN + FAT	PROTEIN + CARB	
Dinner	PROTEIN + FAT	PROTEIN + CARB	PROTEIN + FAT	PROTEIN + CARB	PROTEIN + FAT	PROTEIN + CARB	

WATER INTAKE: ☐ 1/2 gallon (64 oz.) ☐ 1 gallon (128 oz.)

Drink 1 gallon (128 oz.) or at least half of your body weight in ounces of water. A 200lb person should drink at least 100 oz. of water.

WEEKLY REFLECTION

This week's accomplishments:

This week's challenges:

Strategies for next week:

Promises Broken?:

Confess to:
Reassess Promise(s):
Recommit:

CLASSIC CYCLE: SAMPLE WEEK 2 of 4

This week I promise to:

	Monday	Tuesday	Wednesday	Thursday	Friday	Saturday	Sunday
Wake Up	The clock starts as soon as you wake up. Eat breakfast within 30 minutes and meals are spaced every 3 hours thereafter.						
9-Minute Mission	20|10	x reps / x reps / x reps	x reps 2|1 / x reps 2|1 / x reps 2|1	3|0	1x / 2x / 3x	Rest	Rest
Mission Type:	Run Like The Wind Sprintervals	Crazy Eights Super Circuits	Easy Threezies Rapid Rounds	Butt Out Enduro	The Pulse Pounder Step Ladder		
	____total reps / ____total reps / ____total reps	I completed ____ circuits	____rounds / ____rounds / ____rounds	____reps / ____reps / ____reps	I got up to ____reps per circuit		
Shredders			Nasty Nineties				
Intensity:	90 seconds low 90 seconds high	90 seconds low 90 seconds high	90 seconds low 90 seconds high	90 seconds low 90 seconds high	90 seconds low 90 seconds high	Rest	Rest
Overall Duration:	10 minutes	10 minutes	10 minutes	10 minutes	10 minutes		
Morning Weight:	X	X	X	X	X	Weigh In____	X

MEAL TRACKER

	Monday	Tuesday	Wednesday	Thursday	Friday	Saturday	Sunday
	LC	HC	LC	HC	LC	HC	★
Breakfast (within 30 min of waking)	PROTEIN + CARB	PROTEIN + CARB	PROTEIN + CARB	PROTEIN + CARB	PROTEIN + CARB	PROTEIN + CARB	Guilt Free Day
Morning Snack	PROTEIN + FAT	PROTEIN + CARB	PROTEIN + FAT	PROTEIN + CARB	PROTEIN + FAT	PROTEIN + CARB	Enjoy anything you'd like without overdoing it. Aim to intake about 1,000 more calories than normal.
Lunch	PROTEIN + FAT	PROTEIN + CARB	PROTEIN + FAT	PROTEIN + CARB	PROTEIN + FAT	PROTEIN + CARB	
Afternoon Snack	PROTEIN + FAT	PROTEIN + CARB	PROTEIN + FAT	PROTEIN + CARB	PROTEIN + FAT	PROTEIN + CARB	
Dinner	PROTEIN + FAT	PROTEIN + CARB	PROTEIN + FAT	PROTEIN + CARB	PROTEIN + FAT	PROTEIN + CARB	

WATER INTAKE: ☐ 1/2 gallon (64 oz.)   ☐ 1 gallon (128 oz.)

Drink 1 gallon (128 oz.) or at least half of your body weight in ounces of water. A 200lb person should drink at least 100 oz. of water.

WEEKLY REFLECTION

This week's accomplishments:

This week's challenges:

Strategies for next week:

Promises Broken?:

Confess to:
Reassess Promise(s):
Recommit:

CLASSIC CYCLE: SAMPLE WEEK 3 of 4

This week I promise to:

	Monday	Tuesday	Wednesday	Thursday	Friday	Saturday	Sunday
Wake Up	The clock starts as soon as you wake up. Eat breakfast within 30 minutes and meals are spaced every 3 hours thereafter.						
9-Minute Mission						Rest	Rest
Mission Type:	Jackpot Rapid Rounds	Drill Sergeant Step Ladder	The Washboard Enduro	Drop It Like It's Hot Super Circuits	TGIF Sprintervals		
	_____rounds	I got up to	_____reps	I completed	_____total reps		
	_____rounds	_____reps per circuit	_____reps	_____ circuits	_____total reps		
	_____rounds		_____reps		_____total reps		
Shredders			Mighty Minutes				
Intensity:	1 minute low 1 minute high	1 minute low 1 minute high	1 minute low 1 minute high	1 minute low 1 minute high	1 minute low 1 minute high	Rest	Rest
Overall Duration:	15 minutes	15 minutes	15 minutes	15 minutes	15 minutes		
Morning Weight:	X	X	X	X	X	Weigh In_____	X

MEAL TRACKER

	Monday	Tuesday	Wednesday	Thursday	Friday	Saturday	Sunday
	LC	HC	LC	HC	LC	HC	★
Breakfast (within 30 min of waking)	PROTEIN + CARB	PROTEIN + CARB	PROTEIN + CARB	PROTEIN + CARB	PROTEIN + CARB	PROTEIN + CARB	Guilt Free Day
Morning Snack	PROTEIN + FAT	PROTEIN + CARB	PROTEIN + FAT	PROTEIN + CARB	PROTEIN + FAT	PROTEIN + CARB	Enjoy anything you'd like without overdoing it. Aim to intake about 1,000 more calories than normal.
Lunch	PROTEIN + FAT	PROTEIN + CARB	PROTEIN + FAT	PROTEIN + CARB	PROTEIN + FAT	PROTEIN + CARB	
Afternoon Snack	PROTEIN + FAT	PROTEIN + CARB	PROTEIN + FAT	PROTEIN + CARB	PROTEIN + FAT	PROTEIN + CARB	
Dinner	PROTEIN + FAT	PROTEIN + CARB	PROTEIN + FAT	PROTEIN + CARB	PROTEIN + FAT	PROTEIN + CARB	

WATER INTAKE: ☐ 1/2 gallon (64 oz.) ☐ 1 gallon (128 oz.)

Drink 1 gallon (128 oz.) or at least half of your body weight in ounces of water. A 200lb person should drink at least 100 oz. of water.

WEEKLY REFLECTION

This week's accomplishments:

This week's challenges:

Strategies for next week:

Promises Broken?:

Confess to:
Reassess Promise(s):
Recommit:

CLASSIC CYCLE: SAMPLE WEEK 4 of 4 - Slingshot Week

This week I promise to:

	Monday	Tuesday	Wednesday	Thursday	Friday	Saturday	Sunday
Wake Up	The clock starts as soon as you wake up. Eat breakfast within 30 minutes and meals are spaced every 3 hours thereafter.						
9-Minute Mission	3|0	20|10	x reps / x reps / x reps	1x / 2x / 3x	x reps 2|1 / x reps 2|1 / x reps 2|1		
Mission Type:	Monday Funday Enduro	Shoulder Shaker Sprintervals	Lucky Thirteen Super Circuits	Step It Up Step Ladder	Seven Eleven Rapid Rounds	Rest	Rest
	_____reps	_____total reps	I completed	I got up to	_____rounds		
	_____reps	_____total reps	_____	_____reps	_____rounds	Rest	Rest
	_____reps	_____total reps	circuits	per circuit	_____rounds		
Shredders			Thrilling Thirties				
Intensity:	30 seconds low 30 seconds high	30 seconds low 30 seconds high	30 seconds low 30 seconds high	30 seconds low 30 seconds high	30 seconds low 30 seconds high	Rest	Rest
Overall Duration:	20 minutes	20 minutes	20 minutes	20 minutes	20 minutes		
Morning Weight:	X	X	X	X	X	Weigh In_____	X

MEAL TRACKER

	Monday	Tuesday	Wednesday	Thursday	Friday	Saturday	Sunday
	HC	HC	HC	HC	HC	HC	★
Breakfast (within 30 min of waking)	PROTEIN + CARB	PROTEIN + CARB	PROTEIN + CARB	PROTEIN + CARB	PROTEIN + CARB	PROTEIN + CARB	Guilt Free Day
Morning Snack	PROTEIN + CARB	PROTEIN + CARB	PROTEIN + CARB	PROTEIN + CARB	PROTEIN + CARB	PROTEIN + CARB	Enjoy anything you'd like without overdoing it. Aim to intake about 1,000 more calories than normal.
Lunch	PROTEIN + CARB	PROTEIN + CARB	PROTEIN + CARB	PROTEIN + CARB	PROTEIN + CARB	PROTEIN + CARB	
Afternoon Snack	PROTEIN + CARB	PROTEIN + CARB	PROTEIN + CARB	PROTEIN + CARB	PROTEIN + CARB	PROTEIN + CARB	
Dinner	PROTEIN + CARB	PROTEIN + CARB	PROTEIN + CARB	PROTEIN + CARB	PROTEIN + CARB	PROTEIN + CARB	

WATER INTAKE: ☐ 1/2 gallon (64 oz.)   ☐ 1 gallon (128 oz.)

Drink 1 gallon (128 oz.) or at least half of your body weight in ounces of water. A 200lb person should drink at least 100 oz. of water.

WEEKLY REFLECTION

This week's accomplishments:

This week's challenges:

Strategies for next week:

Promises Broken?:

Confess to:
Reassess Promise(s):
Recommit:

TURBO CYCLE

Sample Weeks

TURBO CYCLE: SAMPLE WEEK 1 of 4

This week I promise to:

	Monday	Tuesday	Wednesday	Thursday	Friday	Saturday	Sunday
Wake Up	The clock starts as soon as you wake up. Eat breakfast within 30 minutes and meals are spaced every 3 hours thereafter.						
9-Minute Mission						Rest	Rest
Mission Type:	Stack 'em Up Super Circuits	Push n' Press Enduro	Hard Core Step Ladder	Thigh Master Sprinterval	Five Alive Rapid Rounds		
	I completed _____ circuits	_____ reps _____ reps _____ reps	I got up to _____ reps per circuit	_____ total reps _____ total reps _____ total reps	_____ rounds _____ rounds _____ rounds		

Shredders	Dirty Two-Thirties						
Intensity:	2min30sec low 2min30sec high	2min30sec low 2min30sec high	2min30sec low 2min30sec high	2min30sec low 2min30sec high	2min30sec low 2min30sec high	Rest	Rest
Overall Duration:	5 minutes	5 minutes	5 minutes	5 minutes	5 minutes		

Morning Weight:	X	X	X	X	X	Weigh In_____	X

MEAL TRACKER

	Monday	Tuesday	Wednesday	Thursday	Friday	Saturday	Sunday
	LC	LC	HC	LC	LC	HC	★
Breakfast (within 30 min of waking)	PROTEIN + CARB	PROTEIN + CARB	PROTEIN + CARB	PROTEIN + CARB	PROTEIN + CARB	PROTEIN + CARB	Guilt Free Day
Morning Snack	PROTEIN + FAT	PROTEIN + FAT	PROTEIN + CARB	PROTEIN + FAT	PROTEIN + FAT	PROTEIN + CARB	Enjoy anything you'd like without overdoing it. Aim to intake about 1,000 more calories than normal.
Lunch	PROTEIN + FAT	PROTEIN + FAT	PROTEIN + CARB	PROTEIN + FAT	PROTEIN + FAT	PROTEIN + CARB	
Afternoon Snack	PROTEIN + FAT	PROTEIN + FAT	PROTEIN + CARB	PROTEIN + FAT	PROTEIN + FAT	PROTEIN + CARB	
Dinner	PROTEIN + FAT	PROTEIN + FAT	PROTEIN + CARB	PROTEIN + FAT	PROTEIN + FAT	PROTEIN + CARB	

WATER INTAKE: ☐ 1/2 gallon (64 oz.)   ☐ 1 gallon (128 oz.)

Drink 1 gallon (128 oz.) or at least half of your body weight in ounces of water. A 200lb person should drink at least 100 oz. of water.

WEEKLY REFLECTION

This week's accomplishments:

This week's challenges:

Strategies for next week:

Promises Broken?:

Confess to:
Reassess Promise(s):
Recommit:

This week I promise to:

	Monday	Tuesday	Wednesday	Thursday	Friday	Saturday	Sunday
Wake Up	The clock starts as soon as you wake up. Eat breakfast within 30 minutes and meals are spaced every 3 hours thereafter.						
9-Minute Mission	20|10	X reps	X reps 2|1	3|0	1x 2x 3x		
Mission Type:	Run Like The Wind Sprintervals	Crazy Eights Super Circuits	Easy Threezies Rapid Rounds	Butt Out Enduro	The Pulse Pounder Step Ladder	Rest	Rest
	_____total reps	I completed _____ circuits	_____rounds	_____reps	I got up to _____reps per circuit		
	_____total reps		_____rounds	_____reps			
	_____total reps		_____rounds	_____reps			

			Nasty Nineties				
Shredders							
Intensity:	90 seconds low 90 seconds high	90 seconds low 90 seconds high	90 seconds low 90 seconds high	90 seconds low 90 seconds high	90 seconds low 90 seconds high	Rest	Rest
Overall Duration:	10 minutes	10 minutes	10 minutes	10 minutes	10 minutes		
Morning Weight:	X	X	X	X	X	Weigh In_____	X

MEAL TRACKER

	Monday	Tuesday	Wednesday	Thursday	Friday	Saturday	Sunday
	LC	LC	HC	LC	LC	HC	★
Breakfast (within 30 min of waking)	PROTEIN + CARB	PROTEIN + CARB	PROTEIN + CARB	PROTEIN + CARB	PROTEIN + CARB	PROTEIN + CARB	
Morning Snack	PROTEIN + FAT	PROTEIN + FAT	PROTEIN + CARB	PROTEIN + FAT	PROTEIN + FAT	PROTEIN + CARB	Guilt Free Day
Lunch	PROTEIN + FAT	PROTEIN + FAT	PROTEIN + CARB	PROTEIN + FAT	PROTEIN + FAT	PROTEIN + CARB	Enjoy anything you'd like without overdoing it. Aim to intake about 1,000 more calories than normal.
Afternoon Snack	PROTEIN + FAT	PROTEIN + FAT	PROTEIN + CARB	PROTEIN + FAT	PROTEIN + FAT	PROTEIN + CARB	
Dinner	PROTEIN + FAT	PROTEIN + FAT	PROTEIN + CARB	PROTEIN + FAT	PROTEIN + FAT	PROTEIN + CARB	

WATER INTAKE: ☐ 1/2 gallon (64 oz.)   ☐ 1 gallon (128 oz.)

Drink 1 gallon (128 oz.) or at least half of your body weight in ounces of water. A 200lb person should drink at least 100 oz. of water.

WEEKLY REFLECTION

This week's accomplishments:

This week's challenges:

Strategies for next week:

Promises Broken?:

Confess to:
Reassess Promise(s):
Recommit:

TURBO CYCLE: SAMPLE WEEK 3 of 4

This week I promise to:

	Monday	Tuesday	Wednesday	Thursday	Friday	Saturday	Sunday
Wake Up	The clock starts as soon as you wake up. Eat breakfast within 30 minutes and meals are spaced every 3 hours thereafter.						

9-Minute Mission

Mission Type:	Jackpot Rapid Rounds	Drill Sergeant Step Ladder	The Washboard Enduro	Drop It Like It's Hot Super Circuits	TGIF Sprintervals	Rest	Rest
	_____rounds	I got up to _____ reps per circuit	_____reps	I completed _____ circuits	_____total reps		
	_____rounds		_____reps		_____total reps		
	_____rounds		_____reps		_____total reps		

Shredders — Mighty Minutes

Intensity:	1 minute low 1 minute high	1 minute low 1 minute high	1 minute low 1 minute high	1 minute low 1 minute high	1 minute low 1 minute high	Rest	Rest
Overall Duration:	15 minutes	15 minutes	15 minutes	15 minutes	15 minutes		

Morning Weight:	X	X	X	X	X	Weigh In_____	X

MEAL TRACKER

	Monday	Tuesday	Wednesday	Thursday	Friday	Saturday	Sunday
	LC	LC	HC	LC	LC	HC	⭐
Breakfast (within 30 min of waking)	PROTEIN + CARB	PROTEIN + CARB	PROTEIN + CARB	PROTEIN + CARB	PROTEIN + CARB	PROTEIN + CARB	Guilt Free Day
Morning Snack	PROTEIN + FAT	PROTEIN + FAT	PROTEIN + CARB	PROTEIN + FAT	PROTEIN + FAT	PROTEIN + CARB	Enjoy anything you'd like without overdoing it. Aim to intake about 1,000 more calories than normal.
Lunch	PROTEIN + FAT	PROTEIN + FAT	PROTEIN + CARB	PROTEIN + FAT	PROTEIN + FAT	PROTEIN + CARB	
Afternoon Snack	PROTEIN + FAT	PROTEIN + FAT	PROTEIN + CARB	PROTEIN + FAT	PROTEIN + FAT	PROTEIN + CARB	
Dinner	PROTEIN + FAT	PROTEIN + FAT	PROTEIN + CARB	PROTEIN + FAT	PROTEIN + FAT	PROTEIN + CARB	

WATER INTAKE: ☐ 1/2 gallon (64 oz.)   ☐ 1 gallon (128 oz.)

Drink 1 gallon (128 oz.) or at least half of your body weight in ounces of water. A 200lb person should drink at least 100 oz. of water.

WEEKLY REFLECTION

This week's accomplishments:

This week's challenges:

Strategies for next week:

Promises Broken?:

Confess to:
Reassess Promise(s):
Recommit:

TURBO CYCLE: SAMPLE WEEK 4 of 4 - Slingshot Week

This week I promise to:

	Monday	Tuesday	Wednesday	Thursday	Friday	Saturday	Sunday
Wake Up		The clock starts as soon as you wake up. Eat breakfast within 30 minutes and meals are spaced every 3 hours thereafter.					
9-Minute Mission							
Mission Type:	Monday Funday Enduro	Shoulder Shaker Sprintervals	Lucky Thirteen Super Circuits	Step It Up Step Ladder	Seven Eleven Rapid Rounds	Rest	Rest
	_____reps _____reps _____reps	_____total reps _____total reps _____total reps	I completed _____ circuits	I got up to _____ reps per circuit	_____rounds _____rounds _____rounds	Rest	Rest
Shredders			Thrilling Thirties				
Intensity:	30 seconds low 30 seconds high	30 seconds low 30 seconds high	30 seconds low 30 seconds high	30 seconds low 30 seconds high	30 seconds low 30 seconds high	Rest	Rest
Overall Duration:	20 minutes	20 minutes	20 minutes	20 minutes	20 minutes		
Morning Weight:	X	X	X	X	X	Weigh In_____	X

MEAL TRACKER

	Monday	Tuesday	Wednesday	Thursday	Friday	Saturday	Sunday
	HC	HC	HC	HC	HC	HC	★
Breakfast (within 30 min of waking)	PROTEIN + CARB	PROTEIN + CARB	PROTEIN + CARB	PROTEIN + CARB	PROTEIN + CARB	PROTEIN + CARB	Guilt Free Day
Morning Snack	PROTEIN + CARB	PROTEIN + CARB	PROTEIN + CARB	PROTEIN + CARB	PROTEIN + CARB	PROTEIN + CARB	Enjoy anything you'd like without overdoing it. Aim to intake about 1,000 more calories than normal.
Lunch	PROTEIN + CARB	PROTEIN + CARB	PROTEIN + CARB	PROTEIN + CARB	PROTEIN + CARB	PROTEIN + CARB	
Afternoon Snack	PROTEIN + CARB	PROTEIN + CARB	PROTEIN + CARB	PROTEIN + CARB	PROTEIN + CARB	PROTEIN + CARB	
Dinner	PROTEIN + CARB	PROTEIN + CARB	PROTEIN + CARB	PROTEIN + CARB	PROTEIN + CARB	PROTEIN + CARB	

WATER INTAKE: ☐ 1/2 gallon (64 oz.)   ☐ 1 gallon (128 oz.)

Drink 1 gallon (128 oz.) or at least half of your body weight in ounces of water. A 200lb person should drink at least 100 oz. of water.

WEEKLY REFLECTION

This week's accomplishments:

This week's challenges:

Strategies for next week:

Promises Broken?:

Confess to:
Reassess Promise(s):
Recommit:

FIT CYCLE

Sample Weeks

This week I promise to:

	Monday	Tuesday	Wednesday	Thursday	Friday	Saturday	Sunday
Wake Up	The clock starts as soon as you wake up. Eat breakfast within 30 minutes and meals are spaced every 3 hours thereafter.						

9-Minute Mission						Rest	Rest
Mission Type:	Stack 'em Up Super Circuits	Push n' Press Enduro	Hard Core Step Ladder	Thigh Master Sprinterval	Five Alive Rapid Rounds		

	Monday	Tuesday	Wednesday	Thursday	Friday
	I completed _____ circuits	_____ reps _____ reps _____ reps	I got up to _____ reps per circuit	_____ total reps _____ total reps _____ total reps	_____ rounds _____ rounds _____ rounds

Shredders			Dirty Two-Thirties				
Intensity:	2min30sec low 2min30sec high	2min30sec low 2min30sec high	2min30sec low 2min30sec high	2min30sec low 2min30sec high	2min30sec low 2min30sec high	Rest	Rest
Overall Duration:	5 minutes	5 minutes	5 minutes	5 minutes	5 minutes		

Morning Weight:	X	X	X	X	X	Weigh In _____	X

MEAL TRACKER

	Monday	Tuesday	Wednesday	Thursday	Friday	Saturday	Sunday
	HC	HC	LC	HC	HC	LC	★
Breakfast (within 30 min of waking)	PROTEIN + CARB	PROTEIN + CARB	PROTEIN + CARB	PROTEIN + CARB	PROTEIN + CARB	PROTEIN + CARB	Guilt Free Day
Morning Snack	PROTEIN + CARB	PROTEIN + CARB	PROTEIN + FAT	PROTEIN + CARB	PROTEIN + CARB	PROTEIN + FAT	
Lunch	PROTEIN + CARB	PROTEIN + CARB	PROTEIN + FAT	PROTEIN + CARB	PROTEIN + CARB	PROTEIN + FAT	Enjoy anything you'd like without overdoing it. Aim to intake about 1,000 more calories than normal.
Afternoon Snack	PROTEIN + CARB	PROTEIN + CARB	PROTEIN + FAT	PROTEIN + CARB	PROTEIN + CARB	PROTEIN + FAT	
Dinner	PROTEIN + CARB	PROTEIN + CARB	PROTEIN + FAT	PROTEIN + CARB	PROTEIN + CARB	PROTEIN + FAT	

WATER INTAKE: ☐ 1/2 gallon (64 oz.)   ☐ 1 gallon (128 oz.)

Drink 1 gallon (128 oz.) or at least half of your body weight in ounces of water. A 200lb person should drink at least 100 oz. of water.

WEEKLY REFLECTION

This week's accomplishments:

This week's challenges:

Strategies for next week:

Promises Broken?:

Confess to:
Reassess Promise(s):
Recommit:

This week I promise to:

	Monday	Tuesday	Wednesday	Thursday	Friday	Saturday	Sunday
Wake Up	The clock starts as soon as you wake up. Eat breakfast within 30 minutes and meals are spaced every 3 hours thereafter.						
9-Minute Mission	20|10	X reps / X reps / X reps	X reps 2|1 / X reps 2|1 / X reps 2|1	3|0	1x / 2x / 3x	Rest	Rest
Mission Type:	Run Like The Wind Sprintervals	Crazy Eights Super Circuits	Easy Threezies Rapid Rounds	Butt Out Enduro	The Pulse Pounder Step Ladder	Rest	Rest
	_____total reps	I completed	_____rounds	_____reps	I got up to	Rest	Rest
	_____total reps	_____	_____rounds	_____reps	_____reps per circuit		
	_____total reps	circuits	_____rounds	_____reps			

Shredders			Nasty Nineties				
Intensity:	90 seconds low 90 seconds high	90 seconds low 90 seconds high	90 seconds low 90 seconds high	90 seconds low 90 seconds high	90 seconds low 90 seconds high	Rest	Rest
Overall Duration:	10 minutes	10 minutes	10 minutes	10 minutes	10 minutes		
Morning Weight:	X	X	X	X	X	Weigh In_____	X

MEAL TRACKER

	Monday	Tuesday	Wednesday	Thursday	Friday	Saturday	Sunday
	HC	HC	LC	HC	HC	LC	★
Breakfast (within 30 min of waking)	PROTEIN + CARB	PROTEIN + CARB	PROTEIN + CARB	PROTEIN + CARB	PROTEIN + CARB	PROTEIN + CARB	Guilt Free Day
Morning Snack	PROTEIN + CARB	PROTEIN + CARB	PROTEIN + FAT	PROTEIN + CARB	PROTEIN + CARB	PROTEIN + FAT	Enjoy anything you'd like without overdoing it. Aim to intake about 1,000 more calories than normal.
Lunch	PROTEIN + CARB	PROTEIN + CARB	PROTEIN + FAT	PROTEIN + CARB	PROTEIN + CARB	PROTEIN + FAT	
Afternoon Snack	PROTEIN + CARB	PROTEIN + CARB	PROTEIN + FAT	PROTEIN + CARB	PROTEIN + CARB	PROTEIN + FAT	
Dinner	PROTEIN + CARB	PROTEIN + CARB	PROTEIN + FAT	PROTEIN + CARB	PROTEIN + CARB	PROTEIN + FAT	

WATER INTAKE: ☐ 1/2 gallon (64 oz.)   ☐ 1 gallon (128 oz.)

Drink 1 gallon (128 oz.) or at least half of your body weight in ounces of water. A 200lb person should drink at least 100 oz. of water.

WEEKLY REFLECTION

This week's accomplishments:

This week's challenges:

Strategies for next week:

Promises Broken?:

Confess to:
Reassess Promise(s):
Recommit:

FIT CYCLE: SAMPLE WEEK 3 of 4

This week I promise to:

	Monday	Tuesday	Wednesday	Thursday	Friday	Saturday	Sunday
Wake Up	The clock starts as soon as you wake up. Eat breakfast within 30 minutes and meals are spaced every 3 hours thereafter.						

9-Minute Mission							
Mission Type:	Jackpot Rapid Rounds	Drill Sergeant Step Ladder	The Washboard Enduro	Drop It Like It's Hot Super Circuits	TGIF Sprintervals	Rest	Rest
	_____ rounds _____ rounds _____ rounds	I got up to _____ reps per circuit	_____ reps _____ reps _____ reps	I completed _____ circuits	_____ total reps _____ total reps _____ total reps	Rest	Rest

Shredders			Mighty Minutes				
Intensity:	1 minute low 1 minute high	1 minute low 1 minute high	1 minute low 1 minute high	1 minute low 1 minute high	1 minute low 1 minute high	Rest	Rest
Overall Duration:	15 minutes	15 minutes	15 minutes	15 minutes	15 minutes		

Morning Weight:	X	X	X	X	X	Weigh In _____	X

MEAL TRACKER

	Monday	Tuesday	Wednesday	Thursday	Friday	Saturday	Sunday
	HC	HC	LC	HC	HC	LC	★
Breakfast (within 30 min of waking)	PROTEIN + CARB	PROTEIN + CARB	PROTEIN + CARB	PROTEIN + CARB	PROTEIN + CARB	PROTEIN + CARB	Guilt Free Day
Morning Snack	PROTEIN + CARB	PROTEIN + CARB	PROTEIN + FAT	PROTEIN + CARB	PROTEIN + CARB	PROTEIN + FAT	
Lunch	PROTEIN + CARB	PROTEIN + CARB	PROTEIN + FAT	PROTEIN + CARB	PROTEIN + CARB	PROTEIN + FAT	Enjoy anything you'd like without overdoing it. Aim to intake about 1,000 more calories than normal.
Afternoon Snack	PROTEIN + CARB	PROTEIN + CARB	PROTEIN + FAT	PROTEIN + CARB	PROTEIN + CARB	PROTEIN + FAT	
Dinner	PROTEIN + CARB	PROTEIN + CARB	PROTEIN + FAT	PROTEIN + CARB	PROTEIN + CARB	PROTEIN + FAT	

WATER INTAKE: ☐ 1/2 gallon (64 oz.)   ☐ 1 gallon (128 oz.)

Drink 1 gallon (128 oz.) or at least half of your body weight in ounces of water. A 200lb person should drink at least 100 oz. of water.

WEEKLY REFLECTION

This week's accomplishments:

This week's challenges:

Strategies for next week:

Promises Broken?:

Confess to:
Reassess Promise(s):
Recommit:

This week I promise to:

	Monday	Tuesday	Wednesday	Thursday	Friday	Saturday	Sunday
Wake Up	The clock starts as soon as you wake up. Eat breakfast within 30 minutes and meals are spaced every 3 hours thereafter.						
9-Minute Mission	3|0	20|10	x reps / x reps / x reps	1x / 2x / 3x	x reps 2|1 / x reps 2|1 / x reps 2|1	Rest	Rest
Mission Type:	Monday Funday Enduro	Shoulder Shaker Sprintervals	Lucky Thirteen Super Circuits	Step It Up Step Ladder	Seven Eleven Rapid Rounds	Rest	Rest
	_____reps	_____total reps	I completed _____ circuits	I got up to _____ reps per circuit	_____rounds _____rounds _____rounds		
	_____reps	_____total reps					
	_____reps	_____total reps					

Shredders			Thrilling Thirties				
Intensity:	30 seconds low 30 seconds high	30 seconds low 30 seconds high	30 seconds low 30 seconds high	30 seconds low 30 seconds high	30 seconds low 30 seconds high	Rest	Rest
Overall Duration:	20 minutes	20 minutes	20 minutes	20 minutes	20 minutes		

Morning Weight:	X	_____	X	_____	X	Weigh In_____	X

MEAL TRACKER

	Monday	Tuesday	Wednesday	Thursday	Friday	Saturday	Sunday
	HC	HC	HC	HC	HC	HC	★
Breakfast (within 30 min of waking)	PROTEIN + CARB	PROTEIN + CARB	PROTEIN + CARB	PROTEIN + CARB	PROTEIN + CARB	PROTEIN + CARB	Guilt Free Day
Morning Snack	PROTEIN + CARB	PROTEIN + CARB	PROTEIN + CARB	PROTEIN + CARB	PROTEIN + CARB	PROTEIN + CARB	Enjoy anything you'd like without overdoing it. Aim to intake about 1,000 more calories than normal.
Lunch	PROTEIN + CARB	PROTEIN + CARB	PROTEIN + CARB	PROTEIN + CARB	PROTEIN + CARB	PROTEIN + CARB	
Afternoon Snack	PROTEIN + CARB	PROTEIN + CARB	PROTEIN + CARB	PROTEIN + CARB	PROTEIN + CARB	PROTEIN + CARB	
Dinner	PROTEIN + CARB	PROTEIN + CARB	PROTEIN + CARB	PROTEIN + CARB	PROTEIN + CARB	PROTEIN + CARB	

WATER INTAKE: ☐ 1/2 gallon (64 oz.)   ☐ 1 gallon (128 oz.)

Drink 1 gallon (128 oz.) or at least half of your body weight in ounces of water. A 200lb person should drink at least 100 oz. of water.

WEEKLY REFLECTION

This week's accomplishments:

This week's challenges:

Strategies for next week:

Promises Broken?:

Confess to:
Reassess Promise(s):
Recommit:

YOUR SUCCESS STORY

Throughout the book, I've shared success stories of people who have transformed their lives using my carb-cycling and fitness plans. Now it's your turn! As you start on your journey, feel free to add to this page as you go along—you can have more than one response to many of the prompts. When you've written your story, let us know about it! We love to hear from people who have chosen to lose weight and change their lives—and to celebrate in their success!

My Success Story

My starting weight (and date):

....
....
....
....

My moment of clarity:

....
....
....
....

My biggest challenges (and how I faced and overcame them):

....

....

....

....

I was especially proud of myself when:

....

....

....

....

I fell, but didn't fail when:

....

....

....

....

My favorite story of someone helping me along the way:

....

....

....

....

Something important that I learned about myself:

....

....

....

....

My goals for the future:

....

....

....

....

My ending weight (and date):

....

....

....

....

KEEPING THE WEIGHT
OFF FOR LIFE
THE MAINTENANCE PHASE

When it comes to our weight, it seems like most of us are good at two things: gaining it and losing it. If you've gotten to the point where you've reached your goal weight, congratulations! I'm so proud of all you've done! Now your goal should be Maintenance, which can be a whole new challenge because there aren't a lot of guidelines on how to do it. Everyone talks about finding "balance," but nobody has given direction on how to get there . . . until now.

Maintenance is about feeling satisfied. It's also about finding a system of rewards that fulfills your needs on a daily basis. When you are losing weight, food often gets replaced with the good feeling you get from the number on the scale or compliments from your family and friends. So what happens when you are at your goal weight and the compliments slow down? We still need something to look forward to. Welcome to Maintenance . . . and the rest of your life.

Here's the deal. Your body still needs real, whole, natural food. You still need to eat five times a day and drink plenty of water. This is for your overall health and well-being! However, you don't have to deprive yourself for the rest of your life to stay lean. We have found a method that is incredibly simple yet works. In fact, it is so simple, we've summed it all up in three steps:

1. Select Your Cycle.

Select a cycle that works for you. Choose between the Easy and the Fit Cycle—pick the pattern that you feel comfortable with sustaining forever. This cycle will keep you eating five meals every day of good quality food and drinking plenty of water.

The carb cycle I feel most comfortable doing is: _____.

Now let's get to the good stuff. . . .

2. Select Your Rewards.

Declare it ahead of time! Don't blindly wander through the days succumbing to drive-throughs and donuts that Bob from Accounting brought into the office. You'll quickly find yourself right back where you started. Instead, put some thought into it and treat yourself to some quality eats—because you deserve it. Maybe it's some dark chocolate, or a caramel latte from a fancy coffee shop. Think about your five favorite reward foods and list them with the portion you feel comfortable eating.

My favorite reward foods are:

1.

2.

3.

4.

5.

3. Select Your Lifestyle Layers.

We call these regular rewards laced throughout our week "Lifestyle Layers." We simply lay down more and more rewards until we feel totally satisfied throughout our days and feel confident that we can make it a lifestyle. Don't worry about rewards on high- or low-carb days anymore, just keep the carb-cycling pattern consistent and lay down rewards where *you* feel that you need them. Whatever you do, DO NOT select to reward yourself less than what will satisfy you. This will lead to feelings of deprivation and inevitably going back to old destructive eating patterns. The *right* way to do Maintenance is to keep laying down lifestyle layers until you feel satisfied!

Once a week: If you felt totally satisfied while carb cycling and can maintain that pattern indefinitely, then feel free to indulge in your reward day once a week . . . for life!

Twice a week: Pick two days to reward yourself. Try splitting them up, like Wednesday and Sunday.

Every other day: Similar to the reward plan on the Easy Cycle—if you can't have it today, you can always have it tomorrow!

Once a day: First thing in the morning or later in the day, a daily reward gives us something to look forward to always.

Once you've selected the Lifestyle Layer that works best for you, give yourself an acceptable weight range to stay within—say plus or minus ten pounds.

My upper range limit for Maintenance is: _____.

My lower range limit for Maintenance is: _____.

If at any time during Maintenance you find the number on the scale creeping back up, simply remove a few of the Lifestyle Layers and carb cycle yourself right back down. If you find yourself losing too much weight, follow these steps: Once you find the Lifestyle Layer that works for you, stick with it! Don't add more reward foods to gain the weight back—this can lead you back to the unhealthy eating patterns that made you overweight in the first place. Instead, I want you to add in one hundred calories of smart carbs each day. After a couple weeks, check in to see that you are on track toward your ideal weight.

As you embark on a whole new journey of Maintenance, take to heart the powerful and universal lessons you learned during your weight-loss journey. Keep in mind that nobody does Maintenance perfectly. However, as long as you *unite* with others around you to create a support system, *keep your promises* to yourself, and *fall without failing*, you will always succeed.

Image Credits